Health & Fitness

WALK SLIM

WELCOME to the H&F Walk Slim MagBook. Whether you want to lose weight, increase your fitness or tone up, our 6-week plan will get you in shape. And we'll be with you every step of the way – giving you tips and advice on what to wear, the best moves to boost your training, plus a diet plan to help the pounds fall away.

Cover photography Nigel Riches
Main photography Nigel Riches
Workout photography Danny Bird
Model Jacqueline @MOT
Editor Mary Comber
Writers Lucy Wyndham-Read,
Mary Comber, Eve Boggenpoel
Art editor Claire Punter
Designer Fanni Williams
Sub-editors Sheila Reid, Jo Mattock

MagBook publisher Dharmesh Mistry
Digitial production manager Nicky Baker
Operations director Robin Ryan
MagBook account manager Katie Wood

Senior MagBook account executive
Matt Wakefield
Managing director of advertising
Julian Lloyd-Evans
Newstrade director David Barker
Retail & commercial director
Martin Belson
Publisher Nicola Bates
Group publisher Russell Blackman
Group managing director Ian Westwood
Chief operating officer Brett Reynolds
Group finance director Ian Leggett
Chief executive James Tye
Chairman Felix Dennis

The 'MagBook' brand is a trademark of Dennis Publishing Ltd, 30 Cleveland St, London W1T 4JD. Company registered in England. All material © Dennis Publishing Ltd, licensed by Felden 2012, and may not be reproduced in whole or in part without the consent of the publishers.

Walk Slim Guide ISBN 1-78106-027-4

To license this product, please contact Carlotta Serantoni, +44 (0) 20 7907 6550, carlotta_serantoni@dennis.co.uk. To syndicate this content please, contact Anj Dosaj-Halai, +44 (2)20 7907 6132, anj_dosaj-halai@dennis.co.uk.

While every care was taken during the production of this MagBook, the publishers cannot be held responsible for the accuracy of the information or any consequence arising from it. Dennis Publishing takes no responsibility for the companies advertising in this MagBook. The paper used within this MagBook is produced from sustainable fibre, manufactured by mills with a valid chain of custody. Printed at BGP.

The health and fitness information presented in this book is an educational resource and is not intended as a substitute for medical advice. Consult your doctor or healthcare professional before performing any of the exercises described in this book or any other exercise programme, particularly if you are pregnant, or if you are elderly or have chronic or recurring medical conditions. Do not attempt any of the exercises while under the influence of alcohol or drugs.

Discontinue any exercise that causes you pain or severe discomfort and consult a medical expert. Neither the authors of the information nor the producers nor the distributors of such information make any warranty of any kind in regard to the content of the information presented in this book.

CHΛNGE

TO A SUPERIOR PROTEIN

Diet Protein™ is arguably the most sophisticated diet protein shake available today. Reflex Nutrition have used the latest advances in protein and weight loss science to bring you a product that's specifically designed to help you achieve a healthy, well defined and toned body.

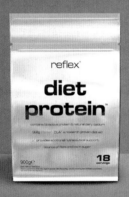

RRP £32.99
900g - 18 x 50g servings

There are many surveys published analyzing the CLA (conjugated linoleic acid) content of foods from around the world which show that intake of CLA is lower than in scientific studies where beneficial health effects are induced.

Research also suggests that in order to obtain the reported health benefits of CLA, supplementation is required.

Reflex Diet Protein™ is the only sports supplement available today that uses a 3.2g daily dose of CLA which is substantiated as an effective dose by research.

Each serving of Reflex Diet Protein™ is packed with additional diet support. Green Tea extract is added for its long standing reputation for aiding dieters.

Diet Protein™ contains no added sugar or maltodextrin. It's perfect for dieters wanting to restrict their carbohydrate content.

Diet Protein™ comes in a variety of mouthwatering flavours, all of which have been up against a taste test panel to ensure that they are the best tasting diet shakes on the market.

Find out more about our products at:

www.reflex-nutrition.com

 Please visit & join our Facebook page at Reflex Nutrition Ltd

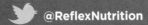 @ReflexNutrition

ecotricity

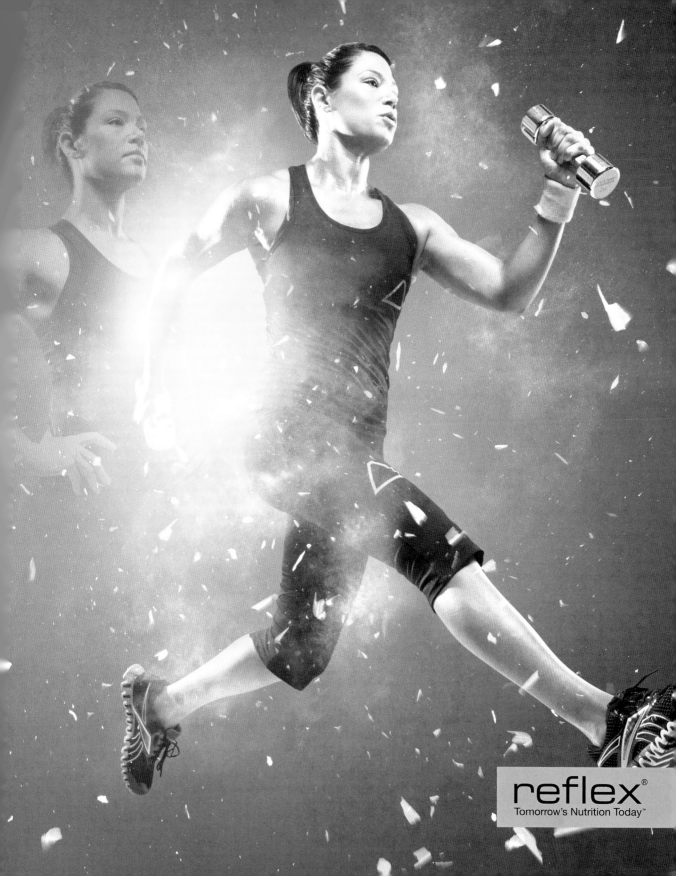

reflex®
Tomorrow's Nutrition Today™

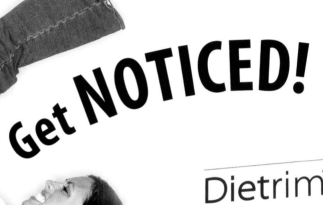

Get NOTICED!

Dietrim®
CAPSULES

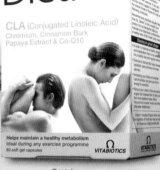

Dietrim®
CLA (Conjugated Linoleic Acid)
Chromium, Cinnamon Bark
Papaya Extract & Co-Q10

Helps maintain a healthy metabolism
Ideal during any exercise programme
60 soft gel capsules   **VITABIOTICS**

Contains
Tonalin CLA
The Shape Of Things To Come™

Achieving the sort of figure that gets you noticed can be a real challenge.

Dietrim® provides advanced dietary support for when you are working hard to maintain a fit and healthy looking body. Each capsule contains 26 ingredients for all round health, including biotin and iodine, which <u>play a role in metabolism and in controlling metabollic rate</u>. It also features Tonalin CLA® (Conjugated Linoleic Acid), a scientifically researched ingredient that is derived from the Safflower plant. Dietrim® helps safeguard your nutritional intake if you are on a dieting programme*, or during exercise, without the need for an additional multivitamin. <u>So let Dietrim® help maintain a healthy you!</u>

Available from Boots, Superdrug, Holland & Barrett, Lloyds pharmacy, Waitrose, pharmacies and health stores or dietrim.co.uk

For more information contact Vitabiotics on 020 8955 2662 or write to us at 1 Apsley Way, London NW2 7HF
Nutritional supplements may benefit those with nutritionally inadequate diets. *This product has not been proven to aid in weight reduction.

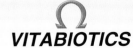

Ω **VITABIOTICS**

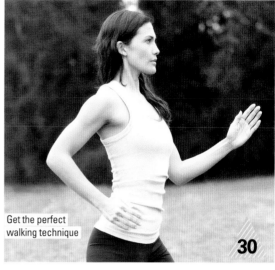

Get the perfect walking technique

30

CONTENTS

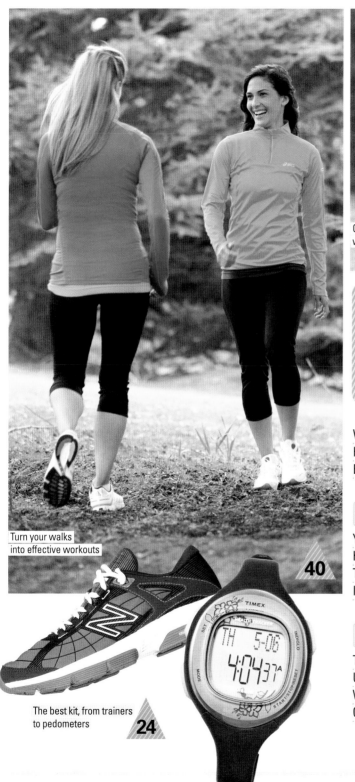

Turn your walks into effective workouts

40

The best kit, from trainers to pedometers

24

〉〉〉〉

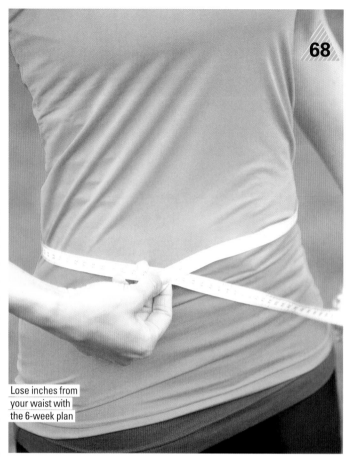

Lose inches from your waist with the 6-week plan

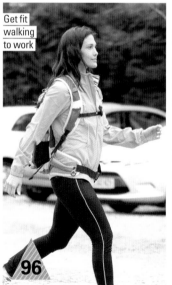

Get fit walking to work

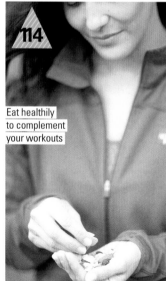

Eat healthily to complement your workouts

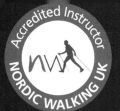
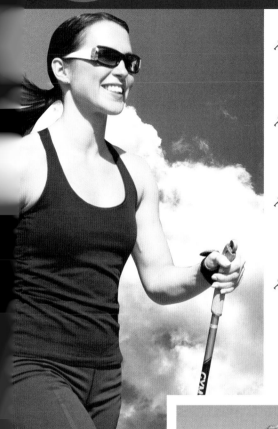
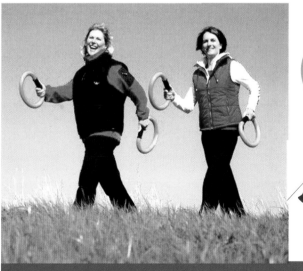

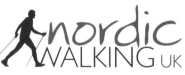

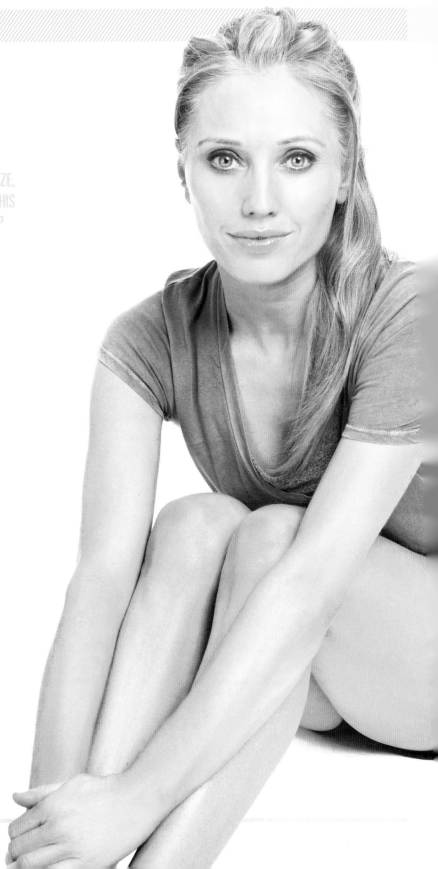

> *WALK SLIM IS IDEAL FOR EVERYONE, SO WHATEVER YOUR SIZE, AGE, WEIGHT OR FITNESS LEVEL, THIS WILL WORK FOR YOU. WE'LL STRIP AWAY BODY FAT AND TONE ALL YOUR TROUBLE SPOTS*

ABOUT:
LUCY WYNDHAM-READ

Lucy Wyndham-Read is a leading women's fitness and weight-loss expert and author of several best-selling fitness books. She produces her own range of audio workouts, DVDs and top-ranking apps. Lucy is also a regular on TV and radio.

During her 15 years' experience in the health and fitness industry she has helped thousands of women lose weight and stay in shape with her creative and effective workouts.

To find more information on Lucy and her products, visit lwrfitness.com.

Welcome

Are you looking for an easy, fun way to lose weight and get fit? Then walk slim is the perfect workout for you! I've designed a 6-week plan that's been tried and tested by my clients. Together, we've come up with a winning formula that's fun to do, simple to follow, easy to fit into your lifestyle and offers fast weight-loss and fitness results. Each week you'll see the pounds and inches drop off, plus feel fitter and healthier. Walk slim is ideal for absolutely everyone, so whatever your size, age, weight or fitness level, this will work for you.

Having helped thousands of women lose weight, I know the one exercise everyone enjoys is walking. It's the most natural form of exercise you can do and offers a whole range of health and fitness benefits. By upping the tempo and using the right technique, you can take your walks from a stroll in the park to a walk-slim workout. I'll make this simple for you by showing you how to walk at speeds that help promote fat loss and inch loss.

Over the next six weeks, I'm going to be your walk-slim personal trainer, motivating you through each week, so you know you're training correctly and to ensure you see super-fast results. Each week, you'll get a new routine to constantly challenge your muscles. I'll also give you 4-minute home workouts to do in between your walking days to supercharge your natural calorie burn, so that we strip away body fat and tone all your trouble spots, from banishing bingo wings to melting away love handles.

Are you ready to walk slim? Then let's get started!

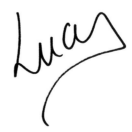

How to use this book

Read this before you start, so you can get the most from your walking workouts!

Not only is walking the easiest, most affordable way to exercise, scientists now know it's one of the best workouts to help you lose weight, get fit and stay healthy. But a casual stroll won't do the trick! To reap the full fat-burning, health-giving benefits, you need to learn the secrets of fitness walking.

Walk Slim offers the expert advice you need to turn your walks into a workout – from tips on technique to a 6-week, walk-slim programme. The book is designed in a progressive format, so we can guide you through the whole journey.

REAP REWARDS
Keeping a workout diary is a proven way to help you stick to your workouts and see more progress. So grab a new journal and start today!

1. PERFECT YOUR TECHNIQUE

Just a few adjustments to the way you walk and the kit you wear will supercharge your walking sessions and transform your body and health. Turn to the first section of this book, 'Get started' (pages 20-37), for your guide to technique, posture, what to wear and how to protect yourself from injury. Getting these essentials in place before you start your workouts will help ensure you reap the best results!

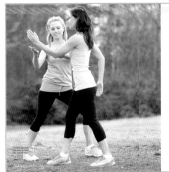

Perfect your techinque

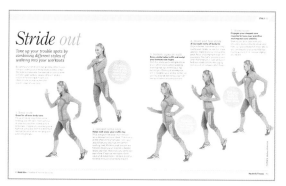

2. TURN YOUR WALKS INTO A WORKOUT

Now you've learnt the basics, it's time to up the pace and start striding. 'Walk fit' (pages 38-57) reveals how often, how far and how fast you need to walk to start seeing results. Discover how to vary your stride to tone up your trouble zones, learn to track your progress with a pedometer and keep your body in top condition with easy warm-up and cool-down sequences.

3. YOUR 6-WEEK PLAN

It's time to walk slim! Follow 'The 6-week plan' (pages 58-91) for a week-by-week programme of progressive walking sessions and workouts that will help you shape up in just over a month. There's plenty of variety to keep you motivated, plus a diary to log all your workouts. You'll also read inspiring stories of women who've followed the plan and transformed their bodies.

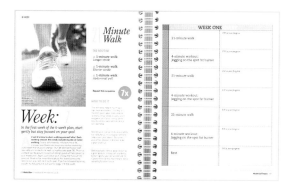

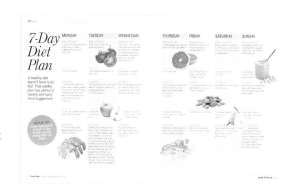

4. WALK FOR LIFE

Now you've seen the benefits that fitness walking has to offer, it's time to find ways to make walking part of your everyday life – and up the challenge! Read the 'Walk on' section (pages 96-111) for ideas on becoming an active commuter, setting up a walking group and training for a charity challenge. There's also a diary of annual walking events, from 5Ks to marathons.

5. EAT SLIM!

Regular exercise, such as walking, is key to helping you lose weight – and ensuring the weight stays off. However, for best results, you need to team your workouts with a healthy-eating strategy. The 'Eat Slim' section (pages 112-123), offers you a 7-day diet plan, plus a wealth of nutrition advice to help you feel your best, as well as see the pounds fall off.

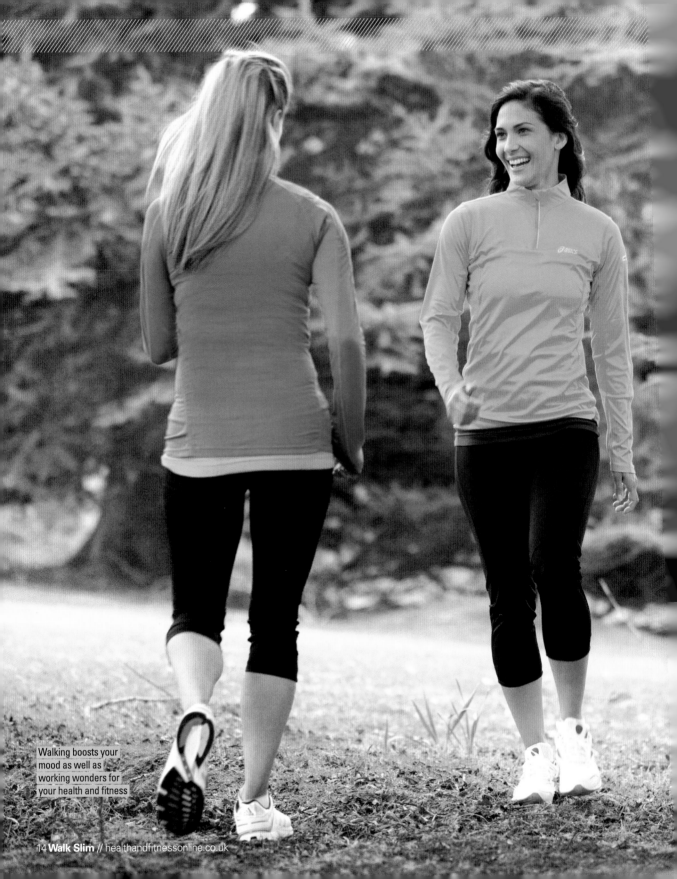

Walking boosts your mood as well as working wonders for your health and fitness

Why walk?

From getting you fit and toned to preventing a whole range of illnesses, here are all the amazing reasons why you should start walking today!

Walking ticks every box when it comes to your health, fitness and wellbeing. Not only is walking the most natural, affordable and convenient exercise you can do, scientists are increasingly realising that walking offers a wealth of benefits for your body and mind – from burning off belly fat to boosting your mood. So much so, the UK Government now recommends that we all walk at least 10,000 steps a day to protect our health and stave off obesity.

While most workouts require expensive kit or costly gym membership, walking is something you can do all year round, anytime, anywhere – for free! Walking fits easily into every lifestyle – you can walk on the way to work, in your lunch hour, while pushing your child through the park or with friends at the weekend. Low-impact and adaptable, walking is also suitable for any age, size and fitness level – everyone can benefit.

Adding more walking into your life can also help you save money.

Research has found that 50 per cent of car journeys are under two miles. Leave the car at home and walk instead and you'll get fit and save money at the same time. Walking is also the perfect stress buster – it's certainly preferable to sitting in traffic!

THE HEALTH BENEFITS

Walking offers a whole host of preventative and curative health benefits for your body and mind. It's been shown to prevent conditions ranging from heart disease to sleep problems, it can help lift depression, reduce high blood pressure and even cut cigarette cravings in those trying to quit smoking. It can be a sociable activity too – walk with a good friend and the miles will fly by as you set the world to rights.

So great are the benefits of daily walking, JoAnn Manson, professor in the department of epidemiology and health at Harvard University describes it as being as close to a magic bullet as you'll find in modern medicine. 'If there was a pill that could lower the risk of chronic disease the way walking ⟩⟩⟩⟩

BEAUTY BENEFITS

Not only does walking do wonders for your body shape, it can also help you look younger!

Walking at a good brisk pace stimulates your circulation, helping nourish your skin cells with oxygen and nutrients and carrying away waste products, cleansing your skin from within. By the end of each walk you'll have a vibrant healthy glow.

Walking also helps you sleep well at night – the key time your body restores and repairs your skin and body.

THE LONGER THE BETTER

Research from the National Walkers' Health Study shows that the further you walk, the more benefits you can reap if you have a condition such as diabetes or high blood pressure. People who completed a walk of 4-6K a week had a lower likelihood of needing anti-diabetic and anti-hypertensive drugs, regardless of how far they walked in total each week.

And the odds of needing these medications were around 30 per cent lower in women who had completed a 6-8K walk each week, compared to those walking less than 4K.

does, people would be clamouring for it,' she says. Here are a few benefits:

Reduces stroke risk

Walking for at least two hours a week could reduce the risk of stroke by 30 per cent. This increases to 37 per cent if you walk at a fast pace, according to a recent study published in the *Journal of the American Heart Association*.

Reduces the risk of diabetes

The odds of developing diabetes decreases the more you walk, if you clock up 15K or more per week, according to research from the National Walkers' Health Study in the US. And, if you already have diabetes, the further you walk the better – the likelihood of needing anti-diabetic drugs was 64 per cent lower in women who walked 45K a week compared with those who walked less than 5K a week.

Improves your blood pressure

Brisk walking strengthens your heart, so it can pump more blood with less effort, helping to reduce high blood pressure. In fact, British research shows that walking is as effective as some drugs in keeping blood pressure levels down. Research from the National Walkers' Health Study found that men and women who walked between 5K and 14K a week were around 24 per cent less likely to need hypertension medication than those walking less than 5K a week.

Reduces your risk of heart disease

A 20-year Nurses' Health Study of 72,000 female nurses found that brisk walking for three hours a week – or just half an hour a day – is associated with a 30-40 per cent lower risk of heart

> BRITISH RESEARCH SHOWS THAT WALKING IS AS EFFECTIVE AS SOME DRUGS IN KEEPING BLOOD PRESSURE LEVELS DOWN

disease. Brisk walking can also reverse the ageing of your heart, according to a year-long study of overweight 50- to 60-year-olds by Washington University in the US. Those who briskly walked for 35-45 minutes a day were found to have hearts that were working as efficiently as those who were in their 30s to 40s.

Keeps your cholesterol levels healthy

Brisk walking helps reduce low-density lipoproteins (LDL) or 'bad' cholesterol which can cause a build up of plaque in your arteries – a major cause of heart attacks.

Protects against hip fracture

Walking helps protect and boost your bones to reduce your risk of brittle bone disease osteoporosis. A study of more than 30,000 men and women aged 20-93 concluded that consistent activity, such as walking, diminishes the risk of hip fracture.

Boosts your mood

It's possible to beat stress and boost your mood with just a 30-minute walk. Walking and other moderate exercise releases happy hormones in the brain called endorphins. These chemicals help to reduce stress, boost the immune system and relieve pain. Recent research carried out by mind. org.uk found that walking outdoors (rather than indoors on a treadmill) is 90 per cent more effective at increasing self-esteem and reducing depression. 》》》

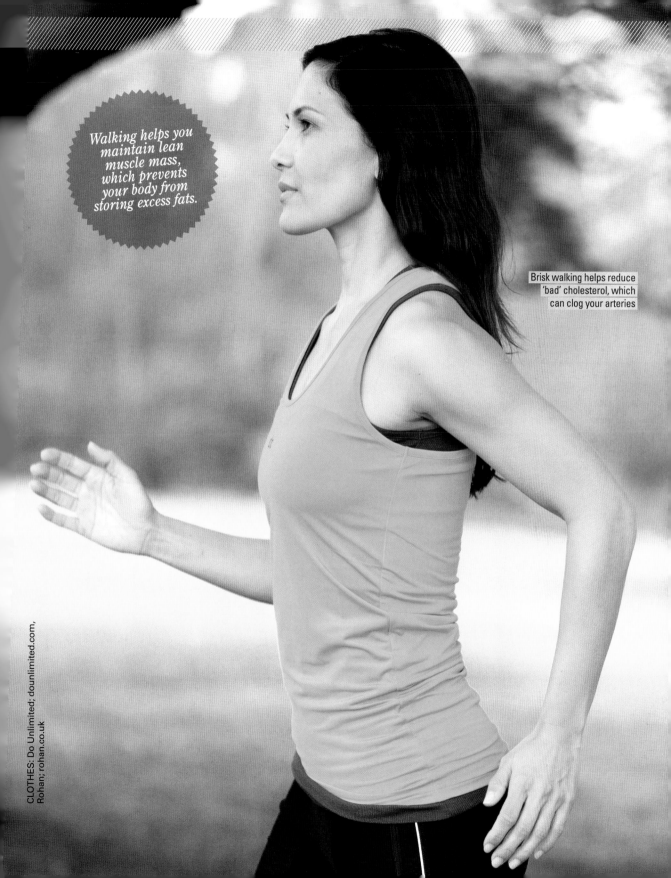

Walking helps you maintain lean muscle mass, which prevents your body from storing excess fats.

Brisk walking helps reduce 'bad' cholesterol, which can clog your arteries

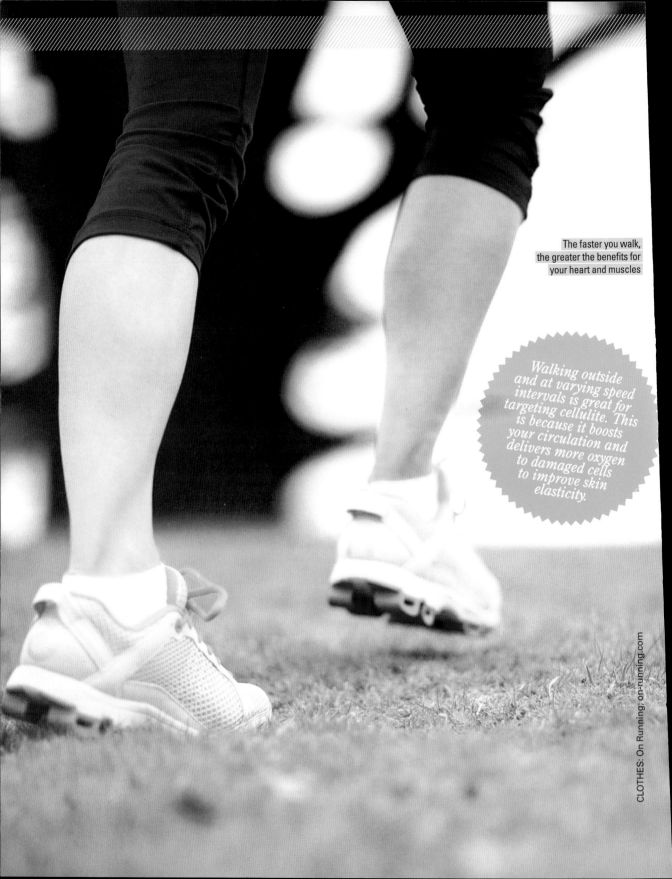

The faster you walk, the greater the benefits for your heart and muscles

Walking outside and at varying speed intervals is great for targeting cellulite. This is because it boosts your circulation and delivers more oxygen to damaged cells to improve skin elasticity.

CLOTHES: On Running; on-running.com

THE FITNESS BENEFITS

Walking is the perfect exercise for weight loss and toning as it engages major muscle groups throughout your body. In fact, walking uses the same muscles as running, but creates less impact on your joints. It's really effective for toning as you work through a bigger ROM (range of movement) than when running. This creates a deeper toning effect in your hips, bottom, abs and even your arms.

Walking also engages your major joints, from your ankles and knees to your hips and shoulders, keeping your body flexible. Researchers at the University of Colorado found that even strolling at a leisurely two miles per hour is enough to help you slim down, if you're usually sedentary. But to get the maximum calorie-burning, fat-busting and toning benefits from your walks, you can't just stroll along! Up the pace and your everyday walks will become an effective workout.

Lose the jelly belly

Can't get rid of that fat around your middle? Scientists have discovered that brisk walking is one of the best ways to burn off stubborn belly fat. Researchers at the University of Virginia in the US compared women who did three shorter, faster-paced walks a week (plus two longer, moderately-paced walks) with a group of women who walked every day at strolling pace. Both groups totalled 12-20 miles a week. Although all the women burned around the same number of calories – 400 per walking workout – those who walked faster lost more than two inches from their waistlines, compared to just half an inch in the slower walkers. They also lost three times more fat from their thighs. Over the course of their 16-week programme, the brisk walkers lost an average eight pounds

each without changing their diets. And the improvements didn't stop there. Walking had a profound effect on reducing fat around their deep organs, linked to diabetes and heart disease. Brisk walking also increases what's called 'afterburn' – the number of calories your body burns after your workout, when you're at rest – by almost 50 per cent compared with a slower, more ambling walking style.

Speed counts

Walking at a faster pace has greater fitness effects because you're pushing your cardiovascular and muscular systems. To reap the benefits, walk at a pace that leaves you breathless – you

> WALKING TWO MILES (3.2K) A DAY, THREE TIMES A WEEK, WILL HELP REDUCE YOUR WEIGHT BY APPROXIMATELY ONE POUND

shouldn't be able to chat non-stop.

So how much walking is enough to get fit? While 10,000 steps a day (about five miles) is the target for health benefits, if walking is the mainstay of your exercise regime, you need to do more than 10,000 steps, incorporating bursts of speed over time.

Varying the terrain you walk on will increase your calorie burn. Walking on softer surfaces, such as grass, uses more energy than walking on concrete; every time your foot hits the ground it creates a small depression so your leg muscles work harder to push forwards. Adding hills also boosts the benefits – on steep inclines, your heart rate can increase by 20 per cent, meaning more calories burned. When you walk downhill, your leg muscles have to work against gravity to slow your descent, which adds toning benefits. ∎

BODY BENEFITS

Follow the walking plans in this book and you'll enjoy the following benefits:

▲ Burn excess body fat.
▲ Lose inches all over.
▲ Reduce cellulite.
▲ Banish your bingo wings.
▲ Melt away your muffin top.
▲ Lengthen and sculpt your legs.
▲ Draw in your waist.
▲ Lose belly fat.
▲ Lift and tone your bottom.
▲ Get your best body ever!
▲ Slow the ageing process.

HAVE A QUICKIE

No time for a long walk? A quick walk can still reap rewards. A study at Loughbrough University discovered three 10-minute walks provided nearly identical increases in fitness as walking continuously for 30 minutes (five days a week). Also, the shorter-distance walkers lost more weight and reported greater decreases in waist circumference than the longer walkers! So just walk when you can and you'll reap the rewards!

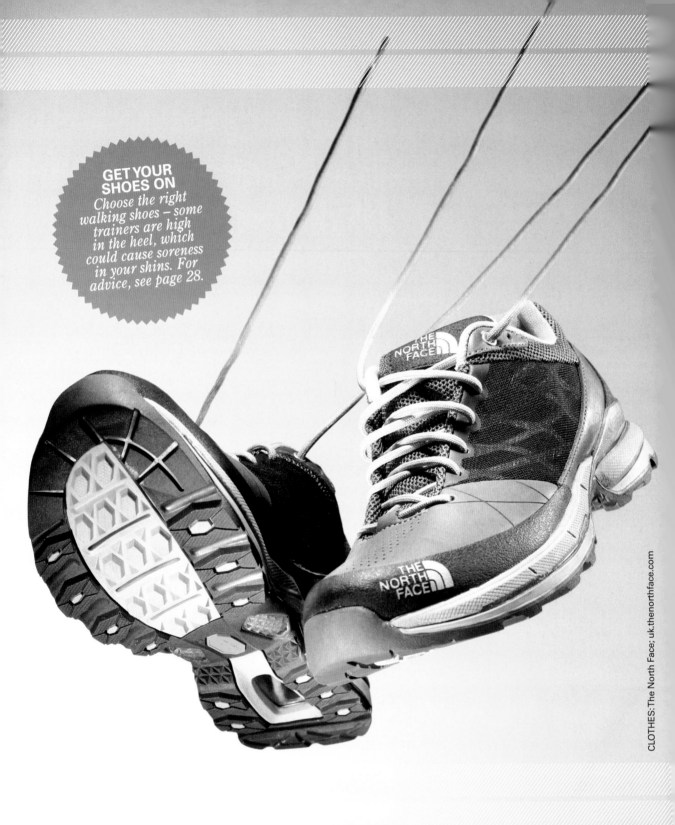

CLOTHES: The North Face; uk.thenorthface.com

GET STARTED

Now you've read about the amazing benefits that walking has to offer, you'll be keen to get started. But first, it's time to learn some key techniques and tips that will help you get more from your walks and prevent any injuries. From the way you stride to the shoes you wear, read on to discover everything you need to know to walk safely and effectively.

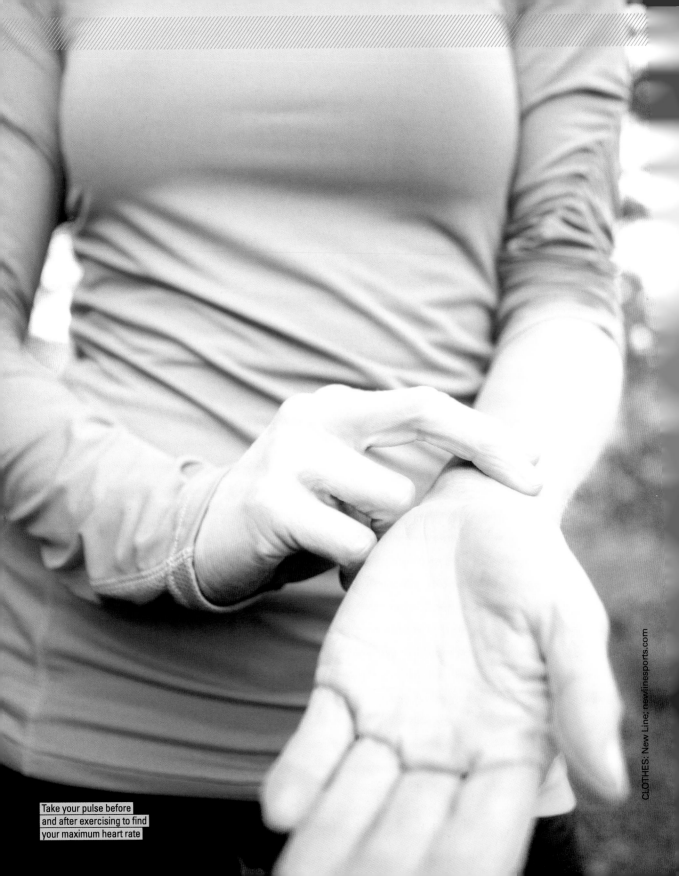

Take your pulse before
and after exercising to find
your maximum heart rate

Walk slim MOT

Make sure you're fit to get in shape with this quick and easy health check

Walking is an incredibly safe form of taking exercise. But if you're new to exercising, recovering from an injury, or have a niggling health problem, it's always best to have a quick health check-up before you start working out.

Read through our health checklist and if you answer yes to any of the questions, see your doctor. It's best to discuss your fitness programme to make sure the exercise you do is in step with your general health.

1 Have you been inactive for a year or more?
☐ Yes ☐ No

2 Have you ever been diagnosed with a heart condition or high blood pressure?
☐ Yes ☐ No

3 Do you smoke or are you a former smoker?
☐ Yes ☐ No

4 Do you have asthma or have you ever suffered from asthma?
☐ Yes ☐ No

5 Is there a history of premature heart problems in your close family (parent or sibling – under 55 in men, under 65 in women)?
☐ Yes ☐ No

6 Do you ever experience chest pain or dizziness during exercise?
☐ Yes ☐ No

7 Have you been diagnosed with a chronic bone or joint problem such as arthritis or osteoporosis?
☐ Yes ☐ No

8 Are you diabetic?
☐ Yes ☐ No

9 Are you trying for a baby, pregnant or have you recently given birth?
☐ Yes ☐ No

10 Do you have a BMI (body mass index) of more than 26?
☐ Yes ☐ No

11 Have you been diagnosed with a chronic condition that may cause problems?
☐ Yes ☐ No

CHECK YOUR HEART RATE

Keeping tabs on your heart rate is a great way to check if you're getting a good workout. Your resting heart rate (RHR) is a good indicator of your health. If it's too high your heart will be working hard to pump blood around your body and if it's too low oxygen isn't being transported efficiently and you may feel light-headed.

The average resting heart rate for adults is between 70 and 90 beats per minute (bpm). Find your pulse by placing two fingers on the inside of your wrist, neck, temple or groin, or by using a sports heart rate monitor. The best time to take your resting heart rate is when you're lying down, having not exerted yourself.

Count your pulse for 15 seconds then multiply the number by four. This is your RHR. Measure your improving fitness levels by timing how quickly it takes you to return to your resting heart rate after each workout.

What to wear

Boost your walks with a few pieces of key kit

The beauty of walking is that you don't need to invest in much kit to get going. The key is that you wear something that's comfortable and visible. However a few pieces of well-chosen kit, such as walking-specific trainers and a sweat-wicking top, can make your walks more enjoyable and effective.

You need to wear items that keep you cool in summer and warm in winter. If you're cold or wet while walking, your posture will suffer. Your shoulders can hunch up and your back rounds as you try to prevent the cold creeping in. So invest in gear that keeps you warm and dry and allows your skin to breathe as you walk. Read on to discover what to buy.

1 TOP
Layers are the key to enjoying your walks. During your workout, your core body temperature will heat up, so it's handy to be able to whip off a layer and tie it around your waist or stash in a backpack. While a regular T-shirt or long sleeve top will do fine, it's best to opt for a breathable base layer in a sweat-wicking fabric. They dry quickly and leave you feeling fresh. In winter invest in a thermal base layer.

2 JACKET
A lightweight jacket is the ideal outer layer – easy to whip off when you warm up. One with pockets is ideal for carrying your essentials such as a mobile

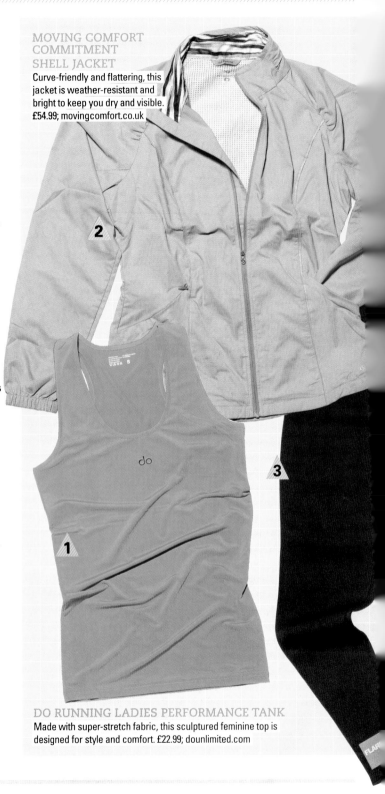

MOVING COMFORT COMMITMENT SHELL JACKET
Curve-friendly and flattering, this jacket is weather-resistant and bright to keep you dry and visible. £54.99; movingcomfort.co.uk

DO RUNNING LADIES PERFORMANCE TANK
Made with super-stretch fabric, this sculptured feminine top is designed for style and comfort. £22.99; dounlimited.com

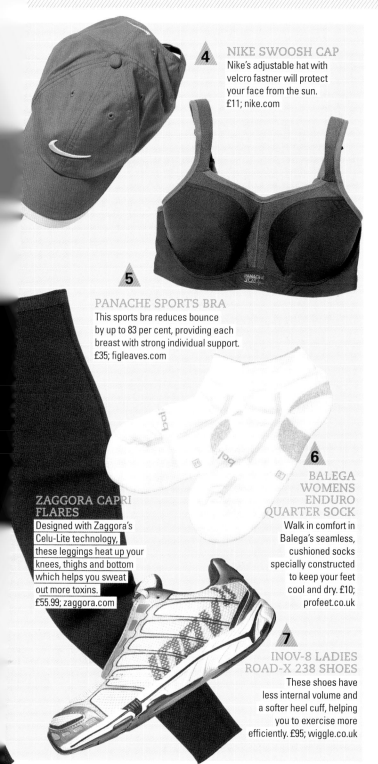

4 NIKE SWOOSH CAP
Nike's adjustable hat with velcro fastner will protect your face from the sun. £11; nike.com

5 PANACHE SPORTS BRA
This sports bra reduces bounce by up to 83 per cent, providing each breast with strong individual support. £35; figleaves.com

ZAGGORA CAPRI FLARES
Designed with Zaggora's Celu-Lite technology, these leggings heat up your knees, thighs and bottom which helps you sweat out more toxins. £55.99; zaggora.com

6 BALEGA WOMENS ENDURO QUARTER SOCK
Walk in comfort in Balega's seamless, cushioned socks specially constructed to keep your feet cool and dry. £10; profeet.co.uk

7 INOV-8 LADIES ROAD-X 238 SHOES
These shoes have less internal volume and a softer heel cuff, helping you to exercise more efficiently. £95; wiggle.co.uk

phone, and high-visibility reflective panels are a bonus if you want to walk after dark. For winter, pick a high-collared, zip-fronted top to keep your neckline warm and prevent hunching your shoulders from the cold.

3 LEGGINGS

A pair of comfortable leggings or shorts will do the trick. But it may be worth getting a pair of running tights, capris or shorts as they're designed to prevent chafing and water-logging. Most have hidden pockets and many have reflective panels. For winter, a pair of lightweight waterproof leggings will keep you dry.

4 CAP

Often overlooked, a sports cap is a good idea if you're training in the heat and sun. It will keep the glare out of your face and protect you from UV damage. A cap can also help prevent heat stroke.

5 SPORTS BRA

For support, comfort and to prevent sagging, a sports bra is a must. Movement in your breasts during exercise can cause the connective tissue of the breast, called the Cooper's ligaments, to sag. Get professionally fitted for your bra but, if that's not possible, look for one that's snug but not so tight it restricts your breathing. Look for seamless or flat-seam designs to prevent chafing.

6 SOCKS

Socks play a vital role providing cushioning and wicking away sweat to prevent blisters. Look for high-tech fabrics and choose double-layered designs to prevent friction. Always wear well-fitting socks – if they're loose they'll rub and can cause blisters.

7 SHOES

You need well-fitting trainers but not a pair of old running shoes. Running trainers are high at the heel to control motion in the rear of the foot but this isn't necessary for walking and makes you overwork your shin muscles which causes soreness. Buy walking trainers (see page 28) or a shoe with a flexible sole that allows you to push through your foot with each stride. To test if they're flexible enough, hold your trainer at either end – you should be able to make it bend slightly without much force. Also look for cushioning in the heel and a breathable upper.

Fit kit

These handy helpers will make your walks that little bit easier

1 WATER BOTTLE
Look for a water bottle with a hole in the middle so that you can hold it easily as you walk. It also works as a mini hand weight which will give you an extra calorie burn.

2 SUNGLASSES
If you're heading out in the sun, it's always best to wear a pair of sunglasses to protect your eyes from the sun's rays. Any UV pair will do but wrap-around runner's glasses are super lightweight and have 100 per cent UVA and UVB protection.

3 MINI RUCKSACK
For safety, it's always best to carry a mobile phone, money, house keys and a water bottle with you, so a bum-bag or small backpack is ideal. Test them out first to find one that doesn't move around or chafe your skin. For longer walks on hot days you could use a hydration pack backpack with a water bladder inside and drinking tube for easy slurps while you're on the move.

4 SPORTS WATCH
This is useful for measuring your walk sessions and training intervals (see page 46), Most will measure your distance travelled, calories burned and average pace.

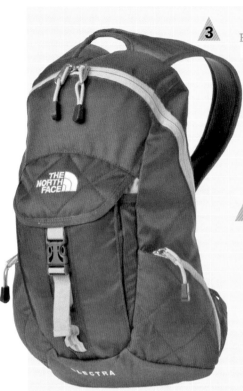

THE NORTH FACE ELECTRA BACKPACK
Ideal for walking with all your essentials, this 12-litre backpack has a large main compartment with several zippable pockets. The wide padded shoulder straps provide extra comfort £39.99; surfdome.com.

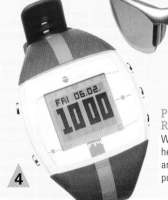

SWEATY BETTY RUN BOTTLE
This easy grip, lightweight and clear water bottle will keep you hydrated as you exercise. £5; sweatybetty.com

RYDERS SHOT SUNGLASSES
These sunglasses have photochromic lenses that adapt to differing light conditions while protecting your eyes. Nose and temple pads hold them in place even if you work up a sweat. £47; snowandrock.com

POLAR FT4 FEMALE HEART RATE MONITOR
Wear it on a brisk walk to monitor your heart levels, making sure you maintain an effective workout. £74.50; polar.fitnessmegastore.co.uk

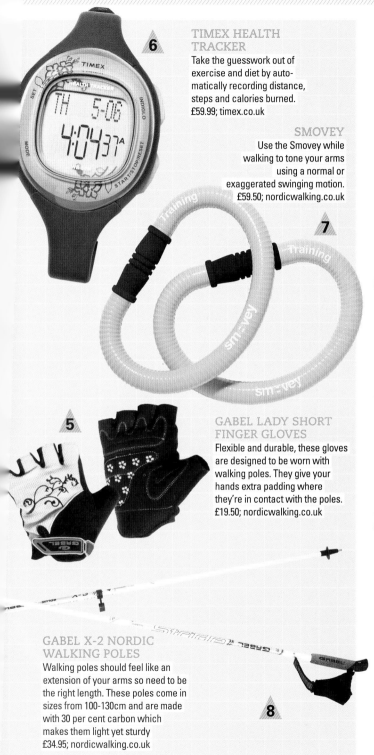

TIMEX HEALTH TRACKER

Take the guesswork out of exercise and diet by automatically recording distance, steps and calories burned. £59.99; timex.co.uk

SMOVEY

Use the Smovey while walking to tone your arms using a normal or exaggerated swinging motion. £59.50; nordicwalking.co.uk

GABEL LADY SHORT FINGER GLOVES

Flexible and durable, these gloves are designed to be worn with walking poles. They give your hands extra padding where they're in contact with the poles. £19.50; nordicwalking.co.uk

GABEL X-2 NORDIC WALKING POLES

Walking poles should feel like an extension of your arms so need to be the right length. These poles come in sizes from 100-130cm and are made with 30 per cent carbon which makes them light yet sturdy £34.95; nordicwalking.co.uk

5 GLOVES

Keeping your hands warm will make your walks more enjoyable in winter. Choose thermal sports-specific fabrics. And if you're walking with poles, wear gloves that are specially designed for them.

6 PEDOMETER

Keep track of the number of steps you're walking with one of these clever gadgets. Choose from basic models which simply measure your steps taken, to more sophisticated numbers that keep track of your progress and log other details such as calories and speed. Styles vary from those you wear around your neck or clip onto your waistband to wrist watches.

7 UPPER BODY WORKOUT

Give your body, especially your arms, a good workout while walking with the Smovey vibrating ring system. These spiral tubes each contain four steel balls and weigh 500g. But when you swing them, the weight increases to 5kg – enough to work up a sweat.

8 NORDIC WALKING POLES

Going for a walk with Nordic walking poles makes you use your upper body as well as your legs. The poles help propel you along so you work harder yet the support they give makes it all feel much easier.

SUMMER SENSE

UV exposure is the number one cause of premature skin ageing and can cause skin cancer so coat yourself with SPF protection (30+) and don't forget the back and sides of your neck and ears. If you can, avoid training when the sun is at its strongest (11am-3pm) and stick to shady routes.

Choose your shoes

From barefoot to tone-up, there's a shoe out there to help you meet your goals

THE NORTH FACE HAVOC

These streamlined and lightweight shoes have shock absorption and heel cushioning for a comfortable stride. £110; thenorthface.com/eu

ASICS GEL-PULSE 3

Versatile and highly cushioned, these help you increase your bounce. £80; asics.co.uk

REEBOK EASYTONE WHITE AND PURPLE REECOMMIT

These trainers help to improve muscle tone through Reebok's Moving Air Technology, which creates micro-instability with every step. £80; next.co.uk

K SWISS BLADE MAX GLIDE

Blade-Light technology provides a perfectly cushioned ride in these high-mileage shoes, making your exercise efficient, yet still comfortable. £95; kswiss.co.uk

TONE UP
Boost walking's benefits by wearing a pair of toning shoes. They have unstable soles that require you to engage your core and tone your legs and bottom.

TRAINING SHOES
Your standard walk-slim shoe of choice should be a lightweight trainer with a flexible sole.

NEW BALANCE 813

This stylish cross-training shoe is lightweight and designed to prevent the numbness often experienced when doing cardio, helping you on your way to fitness. £59.99; newbalance.co.uk

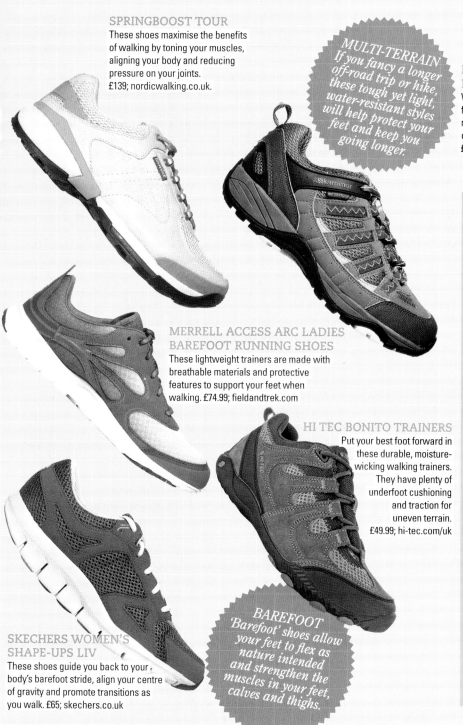

SPRINGBOOST TOUR
These shoes maximise the benefits of walking by toning your muscles, aligning your body and reducing pressure on your joints.
£139; nordicwalking.co.uk.

MULTI-TERRAIN
If you fancy a longer off-road trip or hike, these tough yet light, water-resistant styles will help protect your feet and keep you going longer.

KARRIMOR WHIRLWIND II LADIES WALKING SHOES
With enhanced grip and waterproof fabric, these shoes support your midsole, giving you increased comfort as you walk.
£54.99; store.karrimor.com

MERRELL ACCESS ARC LADIES BAREFOOT RUNNING SHOES
These lightweight trainers are made with breathable materials and protective features to support your feet when walking. £74.99; fieldandtrek.com

HI TEC BONITO TRAINERS
Put your best foot forward in these durable, moisture-wicking walking trainers. They have plenty of underfoot cushioning and traction for uneven terrain.
£49.99; hi-tec.com/uk

SKECHERS WOMEN'S SHAPE-UPS LIV
These shoes guide you back to your body's barefoot stride, align your centre of gravity and promote transitions as you walk. £65; skechers.co.uk

BAREFOOT
'Barefoot' shoes allow your feet to flex as nature intended and strengthen the muscles in your feet, calves and thighs.

BAREFOOT WALKING

If you've not tried it already, you've probably heard about the trend for barefoot walking and running. Walking without shoes – or in shoes that mimic barefoot movements – can help exercise your toes and arches to improve shock absorption, strengthen the muscles of your feet and legs and prevent injuries.

It's best to start off gradually if you're not used to walking barefoot. Start with just five minutes as the muscles in your feet may be weak from wearing shoes. Even if you exercise regularly, work up to 45 minutes, three times a week. The safest place to experiment is at home – avoid wearing shoes around the house and in the garden. If you have diabetes or arthritis do check with your GP first as you may need to protect your feet.

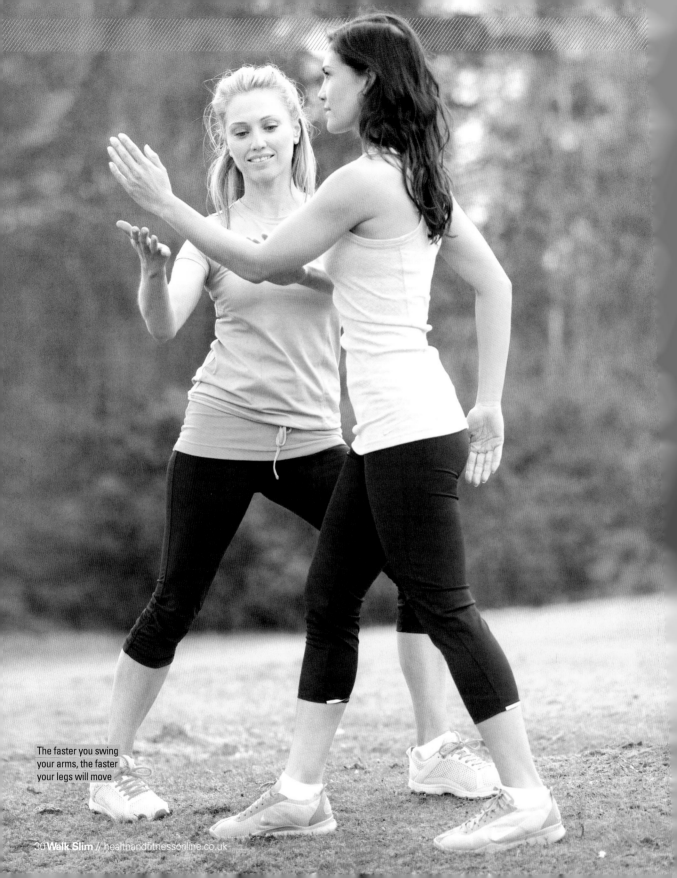

The faster you swing your arms, the faster your legs will move

Perfect your techinque

Walking may be second nature, but perfecting your technique and posture is key to walking slim

Good form is the foundation of your walking plan. Not only will it help you walk faster and longer to reap more benefits, it will help you feel more energetic and look slimmer. Small tweaks to the way you walk can have a big impact on your posture, body shape and weight-loss results. They can also help you walk more comfortably and stay injury free. Follow these guidelines to perfect your stride.

1 Stand tall and create as much distance between your ears and shoulders as possible. This will help prevent hunched shoulders and poor posture. Keep your head in line with your spine and have your chin parallel to the ground – don't tuck in your chin or tilt it back, and this will interfere with your stride.

2 To help maintain correct walking posture, imagine a vertical line from your big toe to the centre of your knee and up to your pelvis.

3 To stabilise your pelvis, keep the front of your pelvis lifted and engage your core by keeping your abdominal muscles slightly contracted. To get the right position, imagine your pelvis contains a bowl of water and aim not to spill any as you walk. This will support your back, flatten your tummy and reduce pressure on your joints.

4 Don't over stride. Take shorter rather than longer strides – this will be better for your joints as well as your posture.

5 With each stride, remember to walk through the whole of your foot. Strike the ground with your heel and roll your foot through to your toes. Focus on pushing off from the ground through all your toes to help activate your glutes and keep your feet aligned. A recent study at the University of Utah found people who walk heel-first use 83 per cent less energy than those who walk on their toes, and 53 per cent less than those who walk on the balls of their feet. 〉〉〉〉

FIND YOUR
MANTRA

Before starting the plan, create a mantra that you say every day for the next six weeks. Your mind is very powerful, and using affirmations can help you achieve your goals and give you an instant burst of inspiration.

Here are some ideas to get you started, simply tailor one of the phrases below to suit your needs and circumstances. Write it out on a piece of paper or print it off and put it where you will see it regularly – on your mirror, on the fridge door, in your car or on your computer screen. You can even send yourself reminders to your phone or computer. The main thing is to keep it in the front of your mind, and to say your phrase to yourself every day.

■ 'I'm going to stick to my walk-slim plan, so I can wear my bikini with confidence this year.'
■ 'No matter what deadlines I have, for the next six weeks I'm going to focus on getting my fittest ever.'
■ 'For the next six weeks, I'm totally engaged in the walk-slim plan, so I can lose those last stubborn pounds.'
■ 'I'm committed to my six-week, walk-slim regime – it will help me complete the 10K Race for Life I'm walking this summer.'

6 For maximum efficiency, use your arms as well as your legs! Walking with straight, rigid arms will impair your technique and make you walk slower. Another common mistake is to allow your arms to swing from side to side rather than backwards and forwards. Instead, bend your arms at the elbow at a 90° angle, and swing them forwards and slightly towards the centre of your body. This will rotate your body, helping tone your waist. Using your arms in this way also helps propel you forward. Basically, the faster you swing your arms, the faster your legs will move.

7 If you're new to power walking, it may be tiring to begin with. If this is the case for you, use your arms in the way described above for five or 10 minutes, then lower your arms and just let them swing naturally to allow them to recover. As soon as you feel rested, raise them again. To build strength in your arms, you could try doing some upper body exercises with dumbbells to increase your endurance.

8 Remember to keep your hands in a relaxed fist – don't clench! If your hands are tight it will create unnecessary tension in your arms and shoulders. It also uses up quite a bit energy – and you want to keep all your energy for walking!

9 To tone up your bottom, concentrate on pushing off with your big toe and little toe after you roll through your heel with each stride. This will help engage your glute muscles more effectively.

10 Try to create some distance between the bottom of your ribcage and the top of your pelvis. This will naturally lengthen your spine. Drop your shoulders and imagine that you are leading from your sternum as you walk, which will keep your chest open and your ribcage slightly forward. This will also make it easier for you to breath more efficiently, and give your muscles more oxygen.

> *USING AFFIRMATIONS CAN HELP YOU ACHIEVE YOUR GOALS AND GIVE YOU AN INSTANT BURST OF MOTIVATION*

11 For optimum breathing technique, breathe in through your nose and out through your mouth. Your nasal passages offer more resistance to the air than breathing through the mouth, and this will help keep your lungs strong and elastic. Breathing out through your mouth will help cool you down. Try to take deep breaths that fill your lungs – short, small breaths won't utilise your lung capacity to the full.

12 Focus your eyes on the ground about five to 10 metres ahead. If you need to look at the terrain closer to your feet, aim to tilt your eyes, rather than your head. If you extend your head forward your body will go out of alignment and you could place excess strain on your neck and shoulders, which will put you off balance and lead to undue fatigue. ■

ARMS
Bend your arms slightly less than a 90° angle. Swing your arms from front to back.

HEAD
Look in front of you, five to 10 metres ahead, not down at the ground.

BACK
Create some space between your lower ribs and your hips, to elongate your spine.

ELBOWS
Don't swing your elbows higher than your sternum (breastbone).

UPPER BODY
Maintain good upright posture through your upper body – imagine you are keeping your shoulders stacked directly above your hips.

CORE
Keep your stomach muscles gently engaged as you walk.

PELVIS
Keep your hips and pelvic area as relaxed as possible, so you're able to walk freely with your legs.

FEET
Concentrate on landing on your heel, rolling through the step and pushing off with your toes.

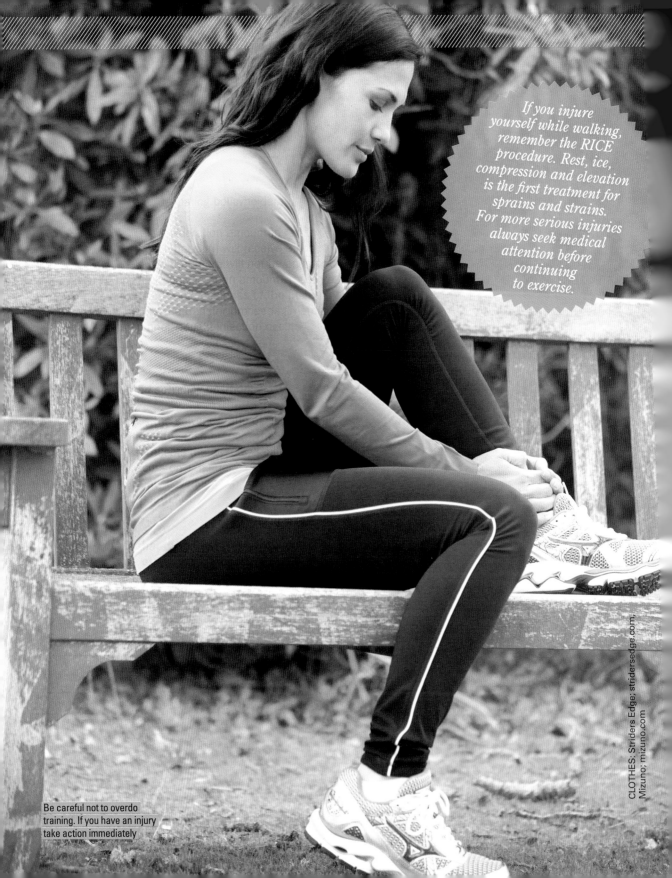

If you injure yourself while walking, remember the RICE procedure. Rest, ice, compression and elevation is the first treatment for sprains and strains. For more serious injuries always seek medical attention before continuing to exercise.

Be careful not to overdo training. If you have an injury take action immediately

Injury proof yourself

Keep your body happy and in top working order with these easy tips and checks

Walking is the most natural exercise you can do yet it's vital to protect yourself from wear and tear. At some point, all exercisers suffer from aches and pains or injury but as long as you're aware of your body and have a balanced approach to training, you can prevent many short-term problems – from sore feet and blisters to niggling knees – turning into more chronic issues.

SAVE YOUR FEET

Always wear well-fitting footwear to support your ankles and create a comfortable cushioning support. Even though walking is low impact, you still get a heel strike when your foot comes into contact with the ground. Invest in your feet, giving them plenty of TLC.

A regular pedicure is a good idea to help prevent any blisters or even ingrown toenails. These are easy to do at home or treat yourself to a pampering session to reward yourself for your weight loss!

LOOK AFTER YOUR KNEES

Your knees take a lot of strain in your day-to-day life so always be kind to them. Walking is low impact, yet be careful, especially if you plan to do lots of cross-country walking.

NEVER SKIP YOUR POST-WORKOUT STRETCH AND TRY TO DO ONE STRETCH SESSION OR CLASS A WEEK. JOIN A YOGA GROUP OR STRETCH IN FRONT OF THE TV

Uneven terrain can lead your knees to extend over the line of your toes which can put extra strain on them. Always keep your knees soft and never lock them out. Be aware of your footing and look out for rabbit holes and well-camouflaged roots along paths in the countryside.

GET YOUR POSTURE RIGHT

Always remember to walk with good posture (see page 30). Hills are great for adding a more intense calorie burn to your workout but you need to adjust your posture to the hill. Keeping a straight back on a hill can cause you to arch your back. To ensure that you have the correct posture for an incline, stop on the hill and check that the heel of your back leg is leading in a straight line all the way to your head.

Be aware of the terrain you're walking on – different terrain presents different challenges. For instance, on uneven cross-country terrain, you activate more muscles to help stabilise yourself on the uneven surfaces.

STRETCH AND PROTECT

Regular stretching is key to keeping your muscles fit, lean and long and to preventing any injuries or tightness.

Never skip your post-workout stretch (see page 52) and try to do at least one dedicated stretch session or class a week. Join a yoga group or do stretches in front of the TV.

Finally, listen to your body and if anything ever feels painful, then stop! 》》》

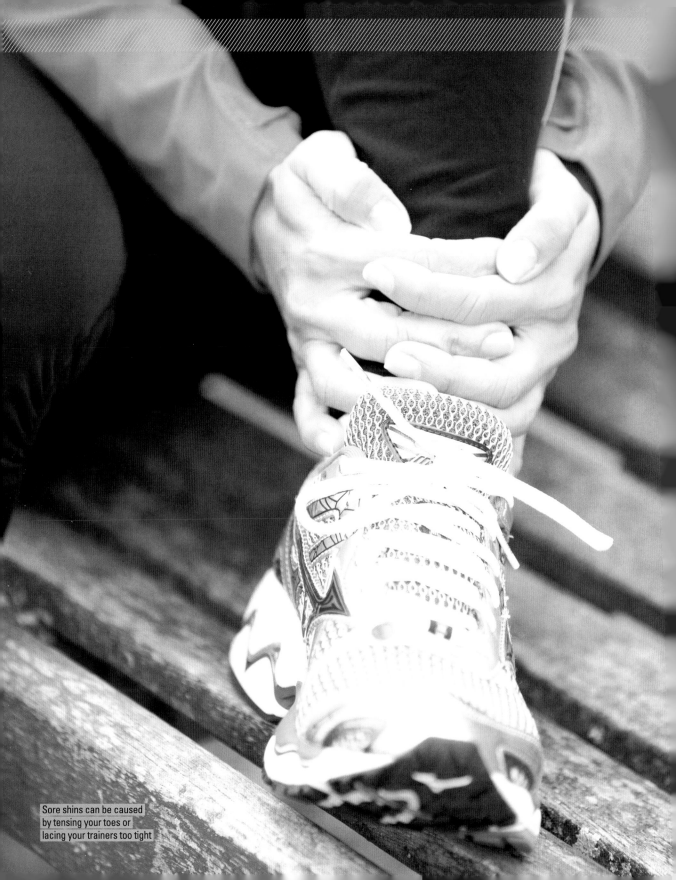

Sore shins can be caused
by tensing your toes or
lacing your trainers too tight

SOLVE YOUR PROBLEMS

Here are simple solutions to three common complaints:

Sore shins

You don't need to be doing many miles to get sore shins. Common causes can be tensing your toes in your shoes or having your trainers laced too tightly. **Solution:** Keep your feet relaxed in your trainers – you should be able to wriggle your toes as you stride. Check the soles of your shoes aren't too rigid – it makes it harder to flex your foot with each stride and distribute the impact right through your foot.

Aching knees

Weak knees and pain around your kneecap can be due to an imbalance between the muscles on the inside and outside of the knee joint. **Solution:** Strengthen the arch of your foot. If your feet are flat with no arch, your foot can roll in and this increases strain on the inside of your knee. To strengthen your arch, roll a golf ball or rolling pin on the floor, trying to pick it up with your foot.

Lower-back pain

This is often due to weak core muscles. Over-striding can also be a culprit. **Solution:** Check your stride length and reduce it if necessary. To improve your core strength and protect your back, pull your tummy in and keep your rib cage down and tucked in. Try pulling your abs in for several strides and then relaxing them for several strides.

STAY SAFE

While losing weight and getting in shape are important, your safety comes first. Here are four ways you can stay safe while walking:

Two's company

It's always safer to walk in a group, especially on dark winter evenings. Join forces with a few friends and drop each other off on the home leg of your walk. Ensure the last person to arrive home texts the rest of you to say she's arrived safely. Alternatively, find a local fitness walking group.

Get visible

When you're choosing new kit, think about visibility and opt for bright, easily visible outer layers or items of clothing with reflective strips.

Carry ID

If you want to travel light, why not invest in an identity wrist tag. These velcro straps fasten around your wrist

> ⫻ WHEN YOU'RE CHOOSING NEW KIT, THINK ABOUT VISIBILITY AND OPT FOR BRIGHT, EASILY VISIBLE OUTER LAYERS OR ITEMS WITH REFLECTIVE STRIPS ⫻

or on your trainers, detailing your name, address, emergency contact numbers and even a private medical insurance number. Try the CramAlert ID – for more information, visit cram-alert.co.uk

Plan your route

Plan your route and leave a note with your partner or flatmate detailing where you're going and what time you plan to return. Stick to your plan too – don't wander off or stay out too late. ∎

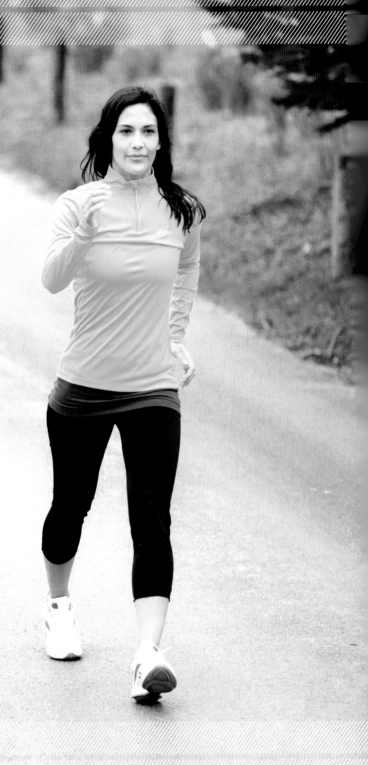

COUNT YOUR STEPS

Aim to walk at least 10,000 steps a day to stay fit and burn fat. A pedometer can help you count them – turn to page 46 for buying advice.

WALK FIT

It's time to hit the road, and you're raring to go. This chapter has tips on how to turn your walks into effective workouts that tone your problem areas while burning calories. But before you set off, make sure you warm up properly to increase flexibility in your joints – and at the end of your walk do cool-down stretches to avoid aches and pains the next day.

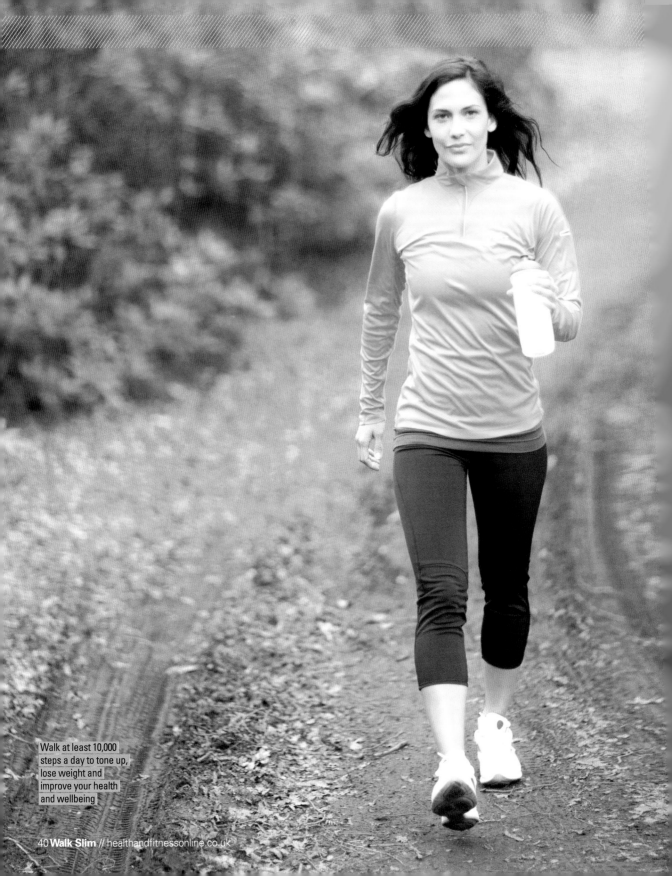

Walk at least 10,000
steps a day to tone up,
lose weight and
improve your health
and wellbeing

Turn your walks into a workout

Take the next step and use your walks to really improve your fitness levels

We all have our own natural pace and speed of walking. But, by upping the speed and varying the way you walk, you can turn each stride you take into a calorie-burning move. Focus on fat-burning, toning your thighs or tightening your tum – read on for tips on all these and how to get the best and fastest results from your walking workouts.

Q. HOW FAR DO I NEED TO WALK?

The Government recommends we aim for 10,000 steps a day to reap health rewards. This may sound a lot but during a 30-minute walk, you can easily take anywhere between 2,000- 6,000 steps and you'll still have the rest of the day to build up to your 10,000 step goal. A good starting point to getting fitter is to establish the average number of steps you currently take a day. Do this by wearing a pedometer for three days. Record the total number of steps you've walked at the end of each day, add them up and divide by three. Here's what your total indicates:

3,000 steps a day – Sedentary.
If you're a complete beginner to fitness, building up from this point will help you start to improve your fitness.

6,000 steps a day – Somewhat active.
This is a level of walking that will help improve your health and prevent ⟩⟩⟩⟩

you from gaining excess weight.

10,000+ steps a day – Active.
You're on target to lose weight and keep super healthy.

Once you've established your baseline number of steps, you can build up your total gradually. Try adding 500 steps a week by building a bit more time into your day for walking – you'll be amazed how quickly the steps add up. The walks in this book are based on time rather than length, but a great walking distance during the week is about two miles. Then, at the weekend, you can head out to tackle longer distances.

Q. HOW FAST DO I NEED TO WALK?

To walk into shape, you need to aim to be walking at between four and five and a half miles per hour. Here's an easy guide to walking paces:

Stroll pace
This is the pace most of us walk at throughout the day – around the house and office for instance. On average, we walk at about two miles an hour. So,

INCREASE YOUR SPEED

The easiest way to improve your walking pace is to set yourself a time trial. Find a small circular walk route and, once a month, challenge yourself to walk it as fast as you can. Record your time and track your progress.

walking at this pace, it would take you about 30 minutes to walk one mile.

Average pace
This is the speed most of us walk if we are outdoors, walking to the office or out shopping, for instance. It's a bit faster – around three miles an hour. So, walking at this pace, it would take 20 minutes to walk one mile.

Walk-slim pace
This faster pace naturally engages your arms. The faster you walk, the more you swing your arms which helps increase your speed. Walk-slim pace is approximately four to five and a half miles an hour. Walking at this pace, you'll complete a mile in about 12 -14 minutes. This difference in intensity and effort pays you a big reward, giving you all the weight loss and toning benefits. As you get fitter, you'll find your speed will increase. The harder you work, the better the results! Try to walk as fast as you can without being so breathless you can't hold a conversation – this is sometimes called the 'talk test'. Walking should be an aerobic exercise to ensure your muscles have sufficient oxygen. If you're gasping for breath, you're doing anaerobic exercise – slow down a little.

Q. HOW OFTEN SHOULD I WALK?

You should be aiming to walk whenever you can. As well as your walking workouts, try to incorporate as much walking into your life as possible. Walk to the shops, walk the kids to school or take a break from your desk and walk at lunchtime – just increase your normal speed to help burn calories. For your

6-week walk-slim plan, I've created a walk-slim diary with all your walks already logged in through the week, to make it easy for you. But as walking is a safe, low-impact exercise, it's great to walk on other days too, if you feel the urge to get out there.

> ❝❝ TRY TO WALK AS FAST AS YOU CAN WITHOUT BEING SO BREATHLESS YOU CAN'T HOLD A CONVERSATION – THIS IS THE 'TALK TEST' ❞❞

Q. WHERE SHOULD I WALK?

Every environment offers a different benefit. Hilly terrain is great as it ups the intensity and gives your legs and bottom a great workout. Cross country is another great challenge as the mixture of terrains means you engage more muscles. Climbing over stiles and gates gives you that extra calorie boost. Beach walking is another great challenge as you have to make more effort moving forwards as the sand doesn't supply you with a solid foundation to propel your heel forwards from. In fact, walking on a sandy beach burns approximately 100 calories per mile. So even while you're on your summer holiday you can stick to your walking plan and keep your mind and body healthy. Closer to home, pavements are a good surface for picking up your speed. Ideally, try to incorporate a range of terrains into your regular walks. ∎

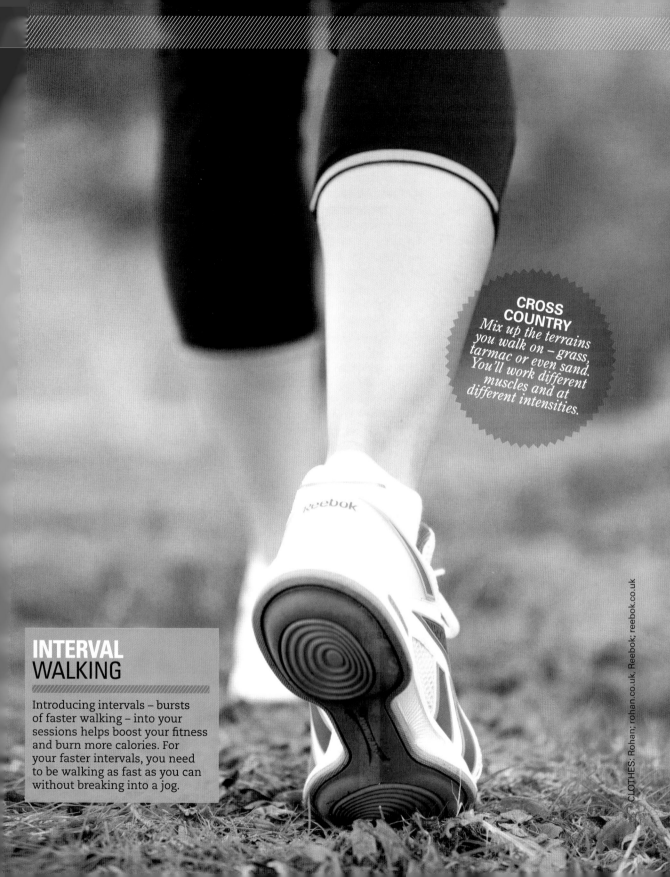

CROSS COUNTRY
Mix up the terrains you walk on – grass, tarmac or even sand. You'll work different muscles and at different intensities.

INTERVAL
WALKING

Introducing intervals – bursts of faster walking – into your sessions helps boost your fitness and burn more calories. For your faster intervals, you need to be walking as fast as you can without breaking into a jog.

Stride *out*

Tone up your trouble spots by combining different styles of walking into your workouts

By varying your stride and incorporating other moves into your walks you can really target problem areas. The walk-slim sessions I've devised for the six-week walk-slim plan combine several different strides – they're all fat burning but each one offers a more intense workout for specific areas of your body.

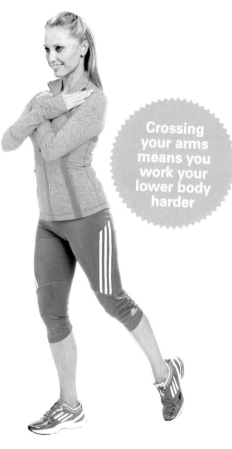

Crossing your arms means you work your lower body harder

1. Brisk walk
Great for all-over body tone
Focus on taking long strides while keeping up a fast pace. Start walking at a normal pace then speed up to a brisk pace. Imagine you're walking on a tightrope and place each foot directly in front of the other while swinging your arms energetically.

2. Crossed arms walk
Helps melt away your muffin top
Walk at a good fast pace, but have your arms crossed over your chest. This means all the effort comes from your hips – you should feel your abs, hips and bottom working hard. Maintain good posture and focus on keeping your shoulders stacked above your hips, then cross your arms over your chest. Focus on walking at a brisk pace while keeping your stride at a normal distance and your upper body straight.

3. Bottom squeeze walk

Every stride helps to lift and sculpt your bottom and thighs

With this stride we're going to shape your bottom muscles by squeezing them tight as you extend your leg behind you. Walking at a brisk pace, aim to lengthen your strides so that, as your leg extends behind you, you can feel your bottom muscles contract.

4. Short and fast stride

A fast walk melts off body fat

With a shorter, fast stride your body has to work harder so you burn more calories. Walking at your normal brisk pace, focus on pumping through with your arms. The faster you pump your arms the faster you'll walk, and you'll find your stride will shorten slightly. Aim to walk at between 4.5-5.5 mph.

5. Waist toner

Engages your deepest core muscles to tone your waistline and improve core stability

Walking at a brisk pace with your shoulders stacked directly above your hips, pull your belly button in as tight as you can towards your spine. Maintain this for a count of 10, release slightly and repeat.

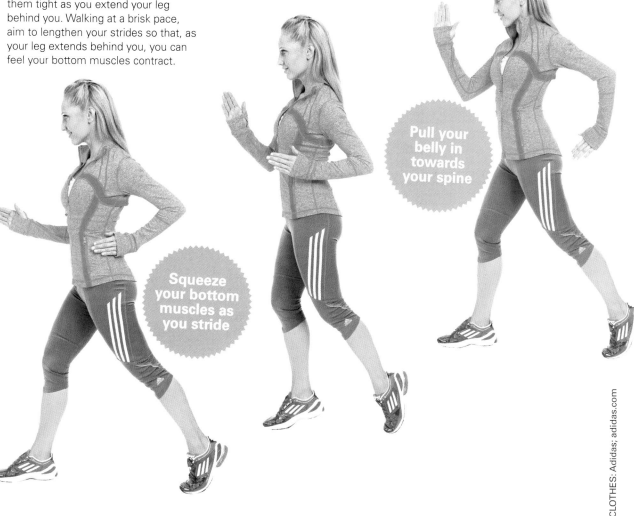

Squeeze your bottom muscles as you stride

Pull your belly in towards your spine

CLOTHES: Adidas; adidas.com

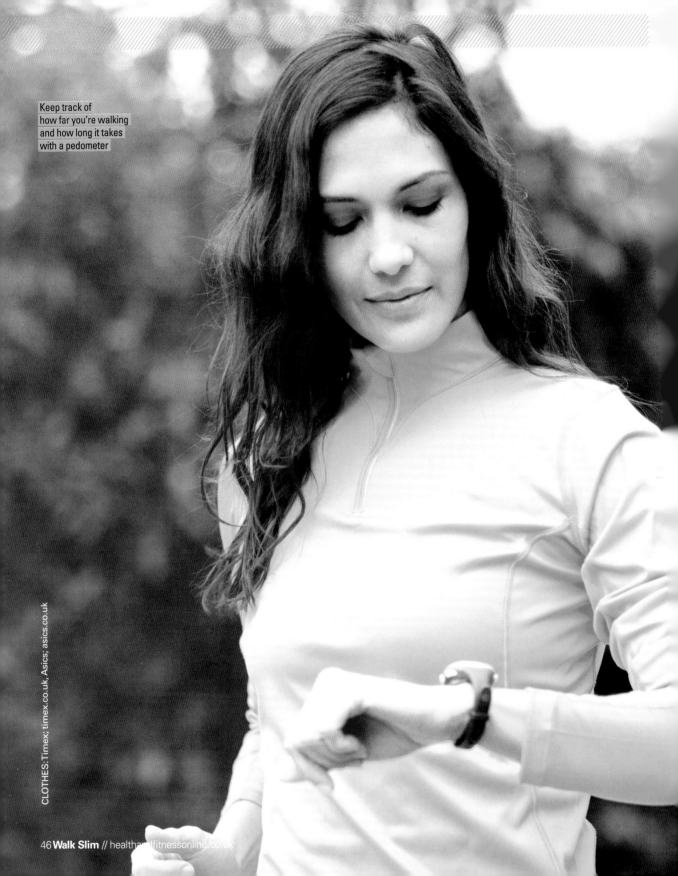

Keep track of
how far you're walking
and how long it takes
with a pedometer

CLOTHES: Timex; timex.co.uk. Asics; asics.co.uk

Using a pedometer

Set and meet your walk-slim goals by tracking the number of steps you walk with a pedometer

A pedometer is a clever gadget that senses your movement and calculates the number of steps you take. It accounts for all step-like movement – not just your walking workouts but walking around the house, the office or climbing stairs, for instance. Pedometers come in different forms – some you can clip onto your waistband, others slip inside your pocket, hang around your neck or are worn as a watch. When you're choosing which pedometer to buy, here are some key points to consider:

HOW TO CHOOSE A MODEL

Some pedometers simply track the number of steps you take. You just clip them on and go, resetting the steps to zero each day. Others can offer more sophisticated features, calculating the time you spend walking, the distance you walk and number of calories you burn, for instance. You may need to programme the date, time and your weight, or calculate and input your length of stride, before you start using it. Some pedometers allow you to upload your data to your computer so you can track your progress. Buy a reputable brand (see box, right) and follow the instruction booklet to ensure you get an accurate reading from your pedometer. Most are reliable at counting steps but it's harder to accurately measure the distance you walk or calories burned. Choose a pedometer that's not too heavy and fits securely to the clothing you usually wear. If you're using a pedometer that clips on your waistband, check your clothes don't affect the reading. Look for a model with a display monitor that you can read in different lighting. Alternatively, turn your smart phone into a pedometer with an app – try iStep for your iPhone or iPod Touch, which calculates distance, speed and calories burned, or Extra Pedometer for Android phones.

USING YOUR PEDOMETER

Establish your baseline steps. Once you've set up your pedometer, wear it throughout the day for three days. Log the total number of steps you take for each of the three days and then divide that total by three. This gives you an average baseline number of steps to build on.

Set step goals. When you know how many steps you take on an average day, you can start to set yourself new targets to build up the distance you're walking. For instance, if you've found you usually walk 5,000 steps a day, aim to add on another 500 steps each day for a week by including some extended periods of walking in your daily routine. You could get off the bus or tube one stop early on your way to and from work to do two 10-minute walks.

TRY THESE

- **Silva ex10 Plus** (£29.99; silva.se) A top-of-the-range model worn around your neck.
- **Tanita PD-724** (£24.99; tanita.co.uk) A versatile pedometer – clip it to your waistband, put it in your pocket or wear it around your neck.
- **Omron Walking Style 1** (£19.95; omron.co.uk) Easily clips to your waistband and clearly shows how many steps you've taken.

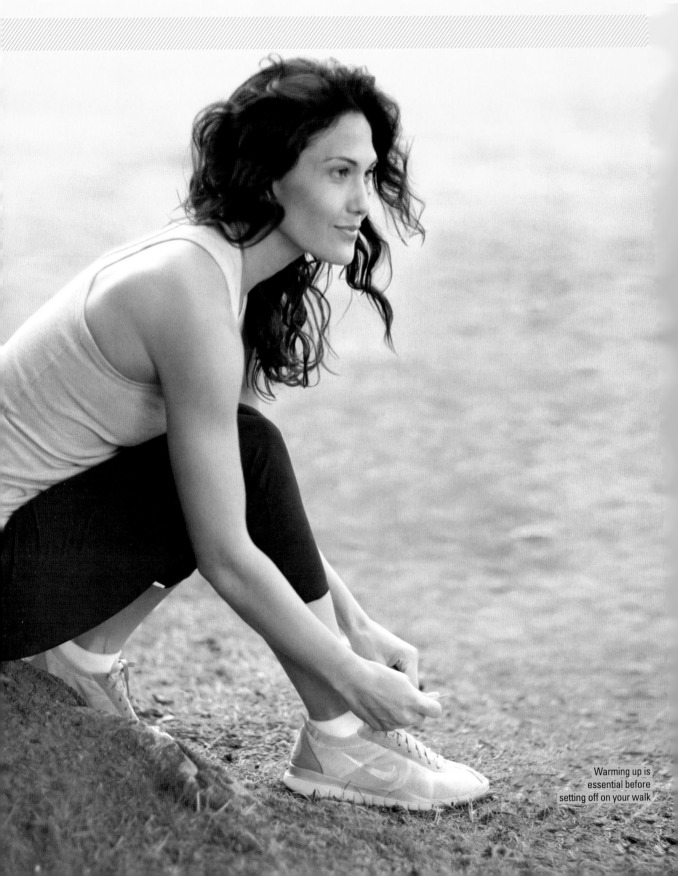

Warming up is
essential before
setting off on your walk

Warm up to walk

Get ready to walk with these easy moves

very walk should consist of the following elements – a dynamic warm-up with flexibility exercises, the walk, a cool-down with final stretches. You might think there's no need to warm up if you're heading out for a walking session, but it's vital to help prevent injury and increase flexibility in your joints and muscles so you feel less stiff and have a greater range of movement.

By warming up, you're gently increasing your body's natural core temperature. It's like switching on a fire

A WARM-UP IS KEY TO HELP PREVENT INJURY AND INCREASE FLEXIBILITY IN YOUR JOINTS AND MUSCLES SO YOU FEEL LESS STIFF

that sends a gentle heat through your body to your muscles, ligaments and joints, making them more relaxed and pliable, so you have more mobility and a greater flexibility.

A big mistake is to stretch before warming up. If you're cold, your muscles will not be flexible so going

straight into a stretch can cause strain and tears within the muscles.

You need to do a dynamic warm-up to make your muscles more pliable. This involves exercising at a lower intensity, so take a steady walk for a few minutes. Follow up with the sequence on the next page and the targeted lower body moves below. ⟩⟩⟩

FOCUS ON YOUR LOWER BODY

Wake up your key muscles and joints before setting off.
● **Ankle circles** Lift one foot off the floor and rotate your ankle 10 times. Then switch directions. Repeat with the other leg.
● **Knee circles** Stand with your feet and knees together. With your hands on your knees, rotate them in a clockwise circle 10 times before changing direction.
● **Hip circles** Make big clockwise circles with your hips. Do this 10 times in both directions.

CLOTHES: Nike; nikestore.com, Rohan; rohan.co.uk

Your *dynamic warm-up*

This easy sequence will raise your pulse and get your body supple

Walk at your normal pace for 30 seconds. Then increase your pace for a couple of minutes. If it's a very cold day you may want to spend a little longer on this until you feel warm. You can also do the following pre-walk warm-up moves, especially before your 4-minute indoor workouts, see page 70.

Lift your knees to get your blood pumping through your body

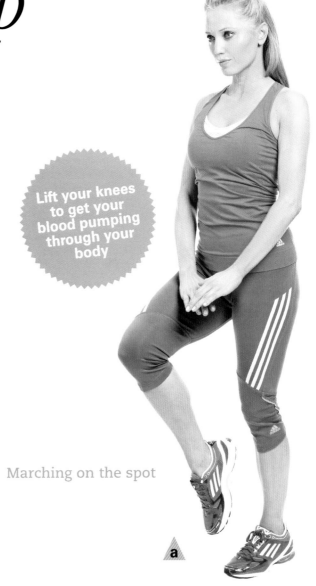

Marching on the spot

a

Circle your arms above your head to get yourself fully warmed up

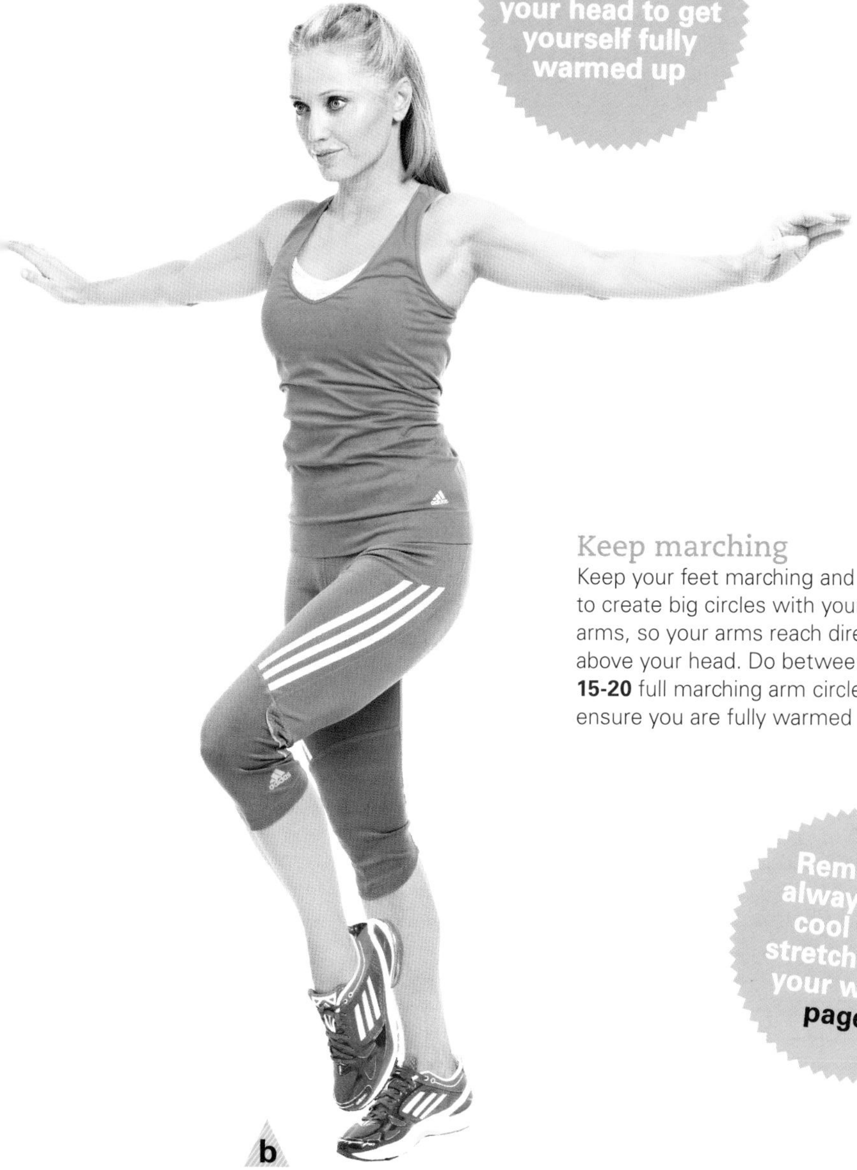

Keep marching

Keep your feet marching and start to create big circles with your arms, so your arms reach directly above your head. Do between **15-20** full marching arm circles, to ensure you are fully warmed up.

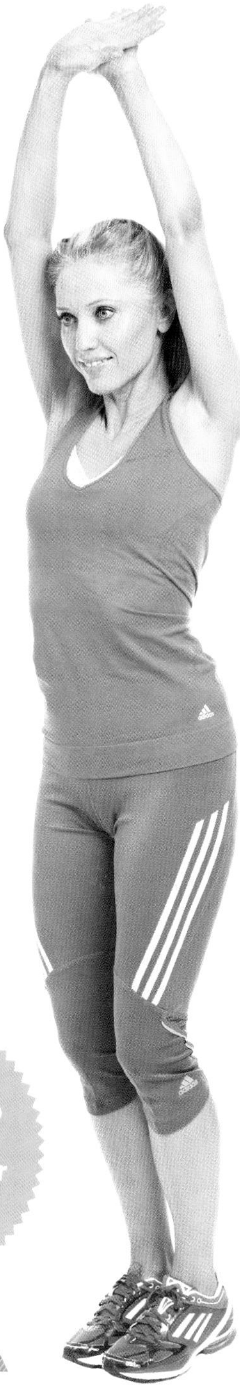

Remember always to do cool down stretches after your walk on page 52

Remember always to do cool down stretches after your walk on **page 52**

b

c

CLOTHES: Adidas; adidas.com

Cool down

Ease out your muscles with these tried and tested moves

Cooling down is vital as it allows your body to come back to its pre-exercise state. If you've been training hard, stopping suddenly can make you feel dizzy, so always spend time slowly reducing your speed to allow your heart rate to fall.

This is also a great time to take some deep breaths to help oxygenate your body. Take a big deep breath in through your nose for four counts, then exhale a big deep breath for four counts. Do this several times while you cool down.

Get ready to put on layers or a jumper as your core body temperature will lower. Now it's time to stretch out your tired muscles to keep them long and lean and help re-align your body and prevent any injuries. Turn the page for some of the best cool-down stretches to use after your walk.

Complementary exercise

When you're following a walking plan, it's a good idea to keep your muscles as flexible and supple as possible. One way to prevent yourself from stiffening up is to do a yoga session once a week. It improves balance, flexibility, coordination, concentration and endurance, while also removing the physical and mental stresses of day-to-

KEEP YOUR MUSCLES SUPPLE AND DO A YOGA SESSION ONCE A WEEK. IT IMPROVES BALANCE, FLEXIBILITY AND ENDURANCE

day life. Yoga rebalances the physical efforts of muscle endurance exercise such as walking and running.

Yoga breathing, called pranayama, is beneficial because it increases lung capacity and helps you find a natural breathing rhythm. 〉〉〉〉

SELF-MASSAGE FOR WALKERS

Foam rolling has many of the same benefits as deep-tissue massage. It can release tension and muscle soreness in the lower back, glutes, hamstrings and calves, so the next time you walk you'll feel fully recovered.

Place the foam roller on the floor and use it to apply pressure to your sore muscles. Roll back and forwards using your body weight. You can buy one from escapefitness.com.

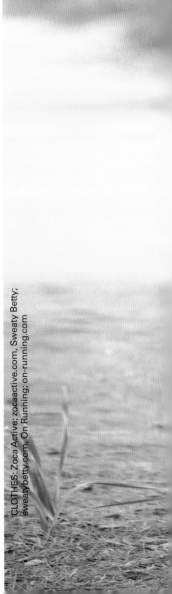

CLOTHES: Zoca Active; zocaactive.com, Sweaty Betty; sweatybetty.com, On Running; on-running.com

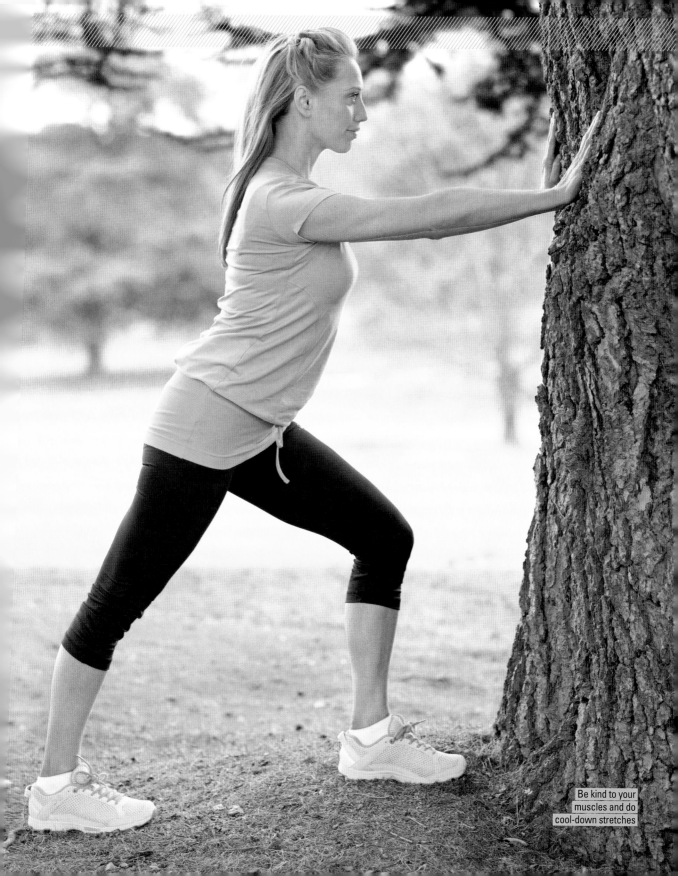

Be kind to your muscles and do cool-down stretches

Cool-down
stretches Do each of these moves to ease out your whole body

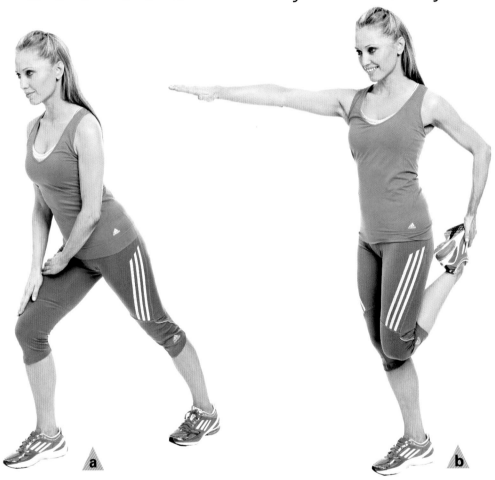

a

b

Lower leg stretch (calf)
Step back with your left leg. Keep the leg straight
and heel down with both feet pointing forwards.
Bend your right leg and rest your hands on this leg,
and feel the stretch in your back leg. Repeat on the
other side. Hold each leg for **10 seconds**.

Quadricep stretch
Stand with good posture, raise your left
leg behind you and hold your foot with
your left hand while pushing your hips
forwards. Don't lock your supporting leg.
Hold each leg for **10 seconds**.

Hamstring stretch

Bend your right leg and stretch your left leg in front, toes up. Rest both hands on your right leg and feel the stretch all the way through the back of your straight leg. Hold each leg for **15 seconds**.

Tricep stretch

Standing straight, knees slightly bent and tummy pulled in, lift your left arm up and bend it behind your head. Apply gentle pressure with your right hand on your elbow and aim to get your left hand between your shoulder blades. Hold on each arm for **10 seconds**.

Bring your heart rate back to normal with these cool-down stretches

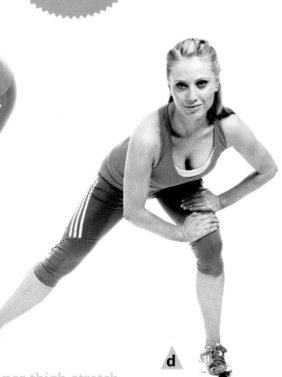

Inner thigh stretch

Extend your right leg out to the side, place both hands on your bent left leg, keeping your tummy pulled in tight and feeling the stretch through the inside of your extended leg. Hold for **15 seconds** then change legs.

c

d

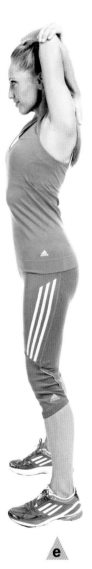

e

〉〉〉〉

Remember, always to do your warm-up on **page 48**

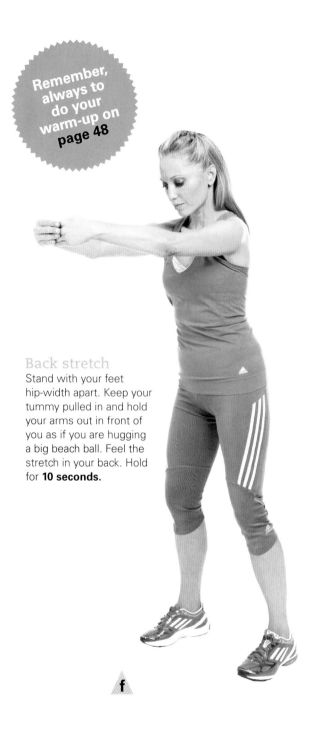

Back stretch

Stand with your feet hip-width apart. Keep your tummy pulled in and hold your arms out in front of you as if you are hugging a big beach ball. Feel the stretch in your back. Hold for **10 seconds.**

f

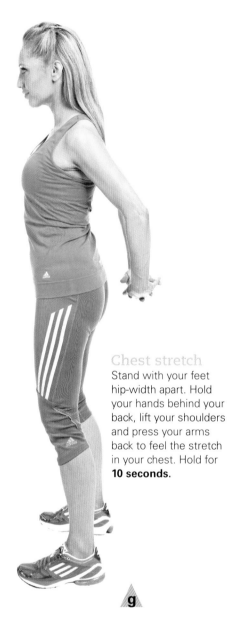

Chest stretch

Stand with your feet hip-width apart. Hold your hands behind your back, lift your shoulders and press your arms back to feel the stretch in your chest. Hold for **10 seconds.**

g

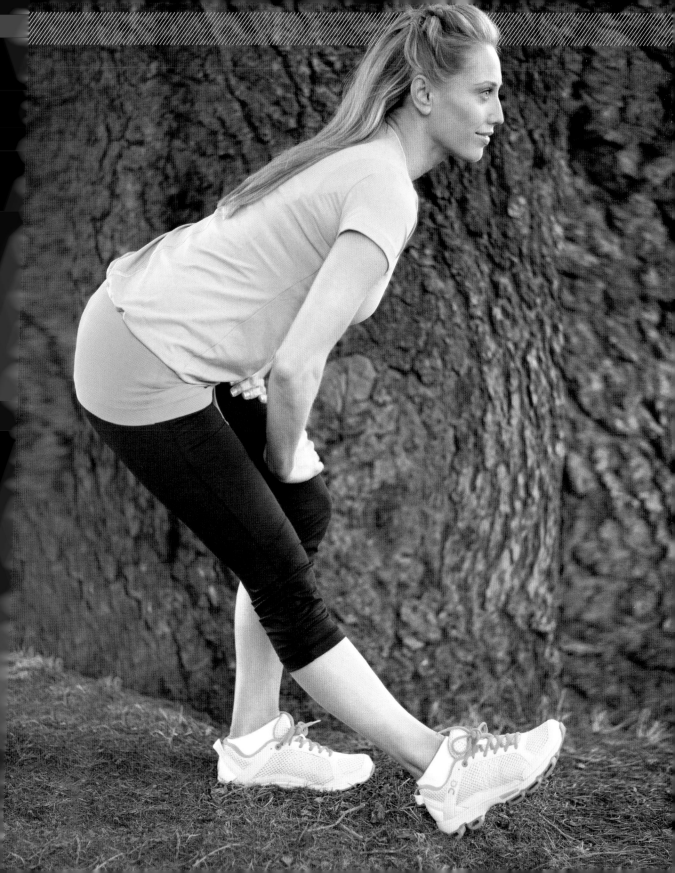

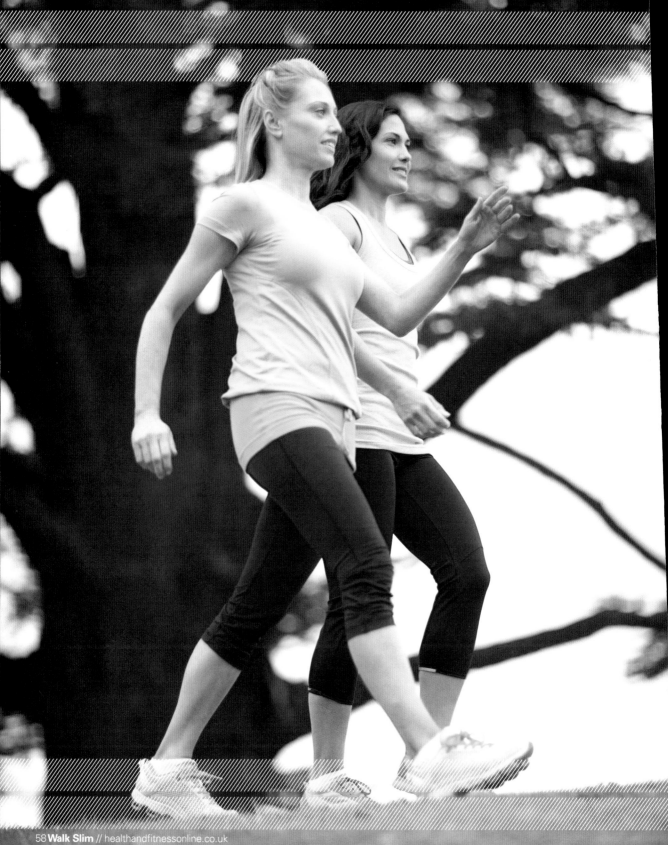

6-WEEK PLAN

Now you know how to turn your walks into a workout, you're ready to start your 6-week walk-slim plan. Whether you want to get fit, lose weight or incorporate more exercise into your daily life, this 6-week plan is just the thing. This perfectly planned combination of walks and easy workouts will not only get you fit and slim, it will also help you feel energised and healthy. Start walking today and you'll be amazed by the results!

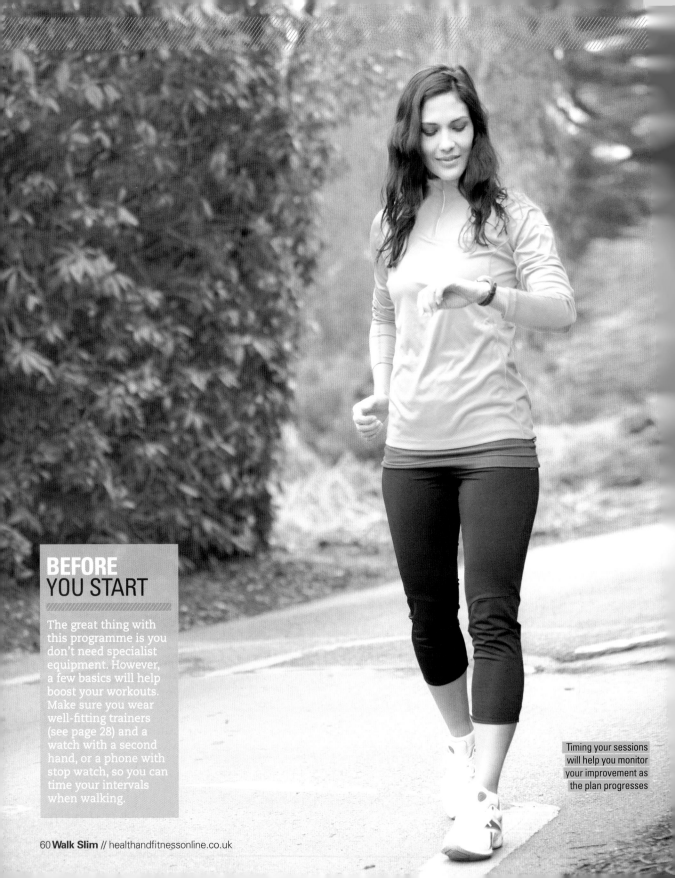

BEFORE
YOU START

The great thing with this programme is you don't need specialist equipment. However, a few basics will help boost your workouts. Make sure you wear well-fitting trainers (see page 28) and a watch with a second hand, or a phone with stop watch, so you can time your intervals when walking.

Timing your sessions will help you monitor your improvement as the plan progresses

How the plan works

This easy 6-week power walking plan will get you fit, slim and toned

So you've got all the tools, techniques and advice you need to start walking into shape. But, to make it even easier for you, I've created a simple but incredibly effective 6-week walk-slim plan.** A combination of power walks and 4-minute workouts, it's super easy to follow and I'll be with you all the way through, offering advice and training tips. From my years of experience, I know that the secret of sticking to your training is all about planning – my clients are more likely to do a workout if they've booked it in their diary – so each week, I've given you a fitness diary with your workouts scheduled in. Just tick off each session once you've completed it.

Your walk-slim sessions are based on interval training – by regularly changing your pace and style of walking, you'll be constantly challenging your muscles. I've also included different styles of walking to help you shape and sculpt

all those problem areas such as that tummy and bottom you're keen to get toned. This variety means each session will fly by and the longest walk is a 30-minute session – short enough to squeeze into your lunch hour! The plan changes each week with a fun, fresh new challenge so you'll never get bored.

QUICK WORKOUTS

The super-speedy 4-minute workouts are designed to raise your metabolism by increasing the amount of calories you burn. These quick workouts create what's known as 'after burn', so for hours after your workout, your body continues to burn off calories – even while you're resting. Each week you'll find a new routine, so the fitter you get, the more I'll be challenging you. I've also chosen moves that will sculpt and shape your waist, arms, legs and bottom. So, if you're ready, let's start and get some amazing results! ⟩⟩⟩⟩

'I did it!'

These inspiring success stories are just the motivation you need to start your walk-slim plan today

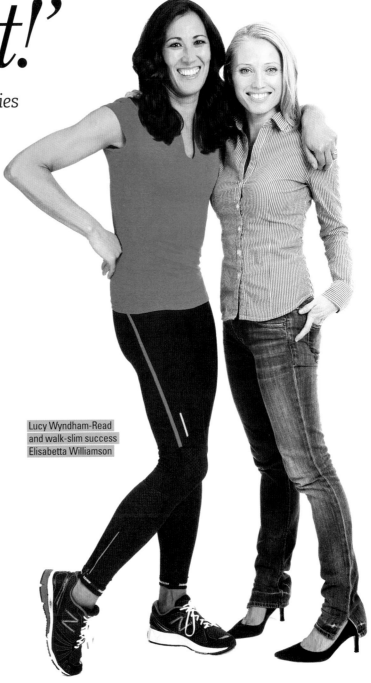

Lucy Wyndham-Read and walk-slim success Elisabetta Williamson

As a personal trainer, I've always known walking is one of the most popular forms of exercise – and one of the best workouts for weight loss. But I was overwhelmed by the response I got when I put out a Facebook request looking for women to trial a new walking weight-loss workout. Women all over the world have now tested my walk-slim plan and reaped the rewards. One woman in the US Navy even told me she's lost more weight doing the plan than she did during her navy fitness training sessions!

The most common feedback I've had from participants is that the walk-slim plan is easy, manageable and enjoyable. Some of the women have struggled for years trying to lose weight. They say this is the first time they've been able to lose weight and keep it off because the plan fits their lifestyle.

Other women emailed me to say how quickly they saw their bum and tums toning up when they started the plan – and we all know that's the best motivation you can have! But the biggest reward for me is that everyone who's tried the plan says they didn't want to stop after six weeks. Here are a few of my favourite success stories.

'I'VE DROPPED TWO SIZES!'

Becki Dicker
Age: 39
Weight lost: 1 stone 6lbs
Inches lost: 8
Dress size dropped: 2

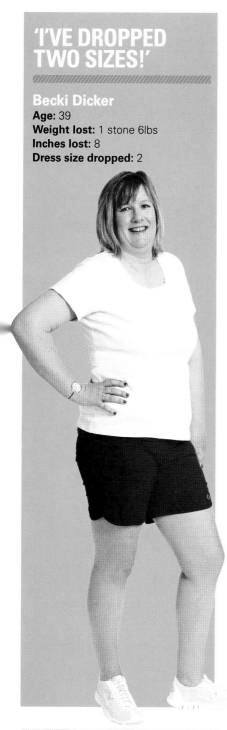

Time for me

'I'm turning 40 in three days' time, so that was the perfect inspiration to try to shed some weight and get my health back on track. I've tried to slim down with various weight-loss programmes before, such as Weight Watchers, but I can honestly say Lucy's walk-slim plan is the most effective I've tried.

'Before I had children I was really active – I used to play hockey to county level so it's not as if I've always been sedentary. But once the children came along all that changed.

'Although I had a weight-loss goal – to lose two stone in four months – I also had another reason for doing the plan. My daughter has been ill for the past 11 years and I'd been neglecting myself, so I felt it was important to do something for myself.

Easy does it

'I did the plan with my husband. We were really strict with ourselves – we followed the diet and workout plans to the letter. I can't stress enough how easy the programme is to do. Because it was so simple, we found sticking to it much easier. After getting the kids up and taking them to school, we did the exercises first thing in the morning. That way we had the rest of the day to ourselves. As we were walking our dogs anyway, incorporating the walking sessions into that time was really easy.

'At first, I used to get tired on the walks, but as the weeks went on, my energy levels improved and it became easier. The 4-minute workouts were also a challenge initially, as they were aerobically demanding for me, but we stuck with it! I think it helped working out with my husband – we bounced off each other – so I'd definitely advise doing the programme with a friend.

New beginnings

'The results I've had have been exceptional. I can't believe the amount I've lost, especially on my waist [almost 6 inches]. I'm a typical apple shape so it's really hard for me to lose weight around my tummy, but now I'm really seeing it shift. And my clothes are

> **I FEEL SO MUCH HEALTHIER NOW, AND MORE MOTIVATED – I FEEL AS IF I COULD TAKE ON THE WORLD**

feeling a lot better having dropped nearly two sizes!

'I continued with the plan after the first six weeks, and I've lost another half stone since this photograph was taken. I now have a totally new outlook on life – I have more energy, I feel healthier and more motivated, and more positive. By about week three, I felt as if I could take on the world!

'We'd been under a lot of stress because of our daughter, but this programme has given me a lifeline. I used to have sleepless nights, but now feel totally rejuvenated – I even feel ready to take on the doctors! I'm now moving on to a 10K plan and looking forward to losing even more weight!'

'I'VE TONED UP ALL OVER!'

Elisabetta Williamson
Age: 45
Results: All-over toning and improved fitness

Group effort

'For me, walking is more about a maintenance regime than losing weight. I think that once you reach a certain age, you tend to have to exercise a little more to maintain your body shape as well as keeping your health in check.

'One of the ways way I stay motivated is by getting a group of mums together so that we can go walking as a group. Once we've dropped the kids off at school, we go walking twice a week. When you're busy with a family there isn't always time to get to the gym, so keeping fit becomes a bit of a balancing act. But walking fits into our schedules really well. Our walks can be anything from 45 minutes to a couple of hours – it depends what we all have on that day, and we decide at the outset how long our walk will be.

'The beauty of exercising together is that if someone walks faster, it acts as motivation to the rest of us. Likewise, if someone is walking a bit slower, you can encourage them to work a bit harder. And if it's a rainy day, for example, it's easy to stay at home with a cup of tea – but we motivate each other to get out. We all realise we're not walking for the sake of walking, we're walking to get fitter – so we power walk.

'Walking with others is a social thing, too. It's nice to know that while having a chat with your friends, you're benefiting physically – you're not just sitting around drinking coffee.

Toning benefits

'I tend to do the 4-minute workouts each day, then every other day, I do circuit training or Pilates. The exercises increase your metabolism and if you do them on a regular basis, you'll definitely become fitter and will burn fat much quicker.

'The thing I've really noticed about following Lucy's plan is that I've not just toned up, but I've also got much more energy. I feel much fitter than I used to. I particularly noticed this

> I HAVEN'T JUST TONED UP, I FEEL MUCH FITTER AND I'VE GOT MUCH MORE ENERGY

when I went on holiday recently – if there were classes such as Pilates on offer, I really enjoyed doing them – I didn't find keeping fit a drag. And, what's more, I also looked forward to coming home and going back into my normal fitness routine.

Have a goal

'If I was to give anyone advice on following the plan, I'd say always have a goal. This will make it easier for you to achieve your aims. I always keep my goals in mind and that helps me stick with the plan. One of the great things about Lucy's programme is that the workouts are easy to fit in – 4 minutes is nothing. You don't even have to do it at home, you can do it at lunchtime, or at work.'

'I'VE TURNED MY HEALTH AROUND'

Farah Isham-Barrett
Age: 41
Weight lost: 1 stone 4lbs
Inches lost: 8
Dress sizes dropped: 3

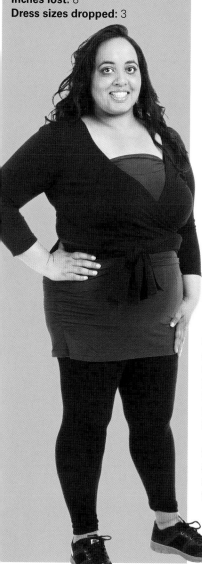

Health alert

'I'd known for some time my health wasn't right. I'd given birth to my first child in January 2011 and had gestational diabetes, and I also have asthma and severe hay fever. Last August, I fell down the stairs and was immobilised for a month. After that, I spiralled into a series of accidents and illness. And, although I knew my weight was at the heart of my problems, I found it hard to focus on weight-loss when I was ill.

'A close friend decided to intervene – she suggested I do the Moonwalk half marathon and introduced me to Lucy. I took my Moonwalk training seriously, but kept getting ill with chest infections and 'flu. Once I started Lucy's plan, though, I no longer fell at these hurdles and kept going. That was the greatest feeling.

Diet help

'Doing the walk-slim plan was really important to me. I want to start singing again as a hobby. I'd also love to do a hike in the Eastern Himalayan foothills, finishing an adventure I started years ago but couldn't finish due to my weight and asthma. I'd also like to climb Mount Fuji in Japan, where I used to live. Most importantly though, as an older first-time mum, I want to be fit and healthy for my son.

'Lucy's plan was really easy to follow. She was very accommodating about sensible changes to the diet to suit my food preferences, and the diet made me very aware of portion sizes.

'Initially, I walked to the station from work instead of getting the bus and then, as I got stronger, I walked home from work (about 9km) once or twice a week. Your body finds a rhythm as you do more walking.

New lease of life

'The results are amazing. Power walking has been a revelation, I've lost weight at a consistent pace, meaning the skin all over my body is in fantastic condition. I'm breathing more easily, and feel so good. Even with

> **POWER WALKING HAS BEEN A REVELATION – I'M BREATHING EASIER AND FEEL SO GOOD**

such a busy life and being mum to a 15-month-old, I'm full of energy – not just physically, but mentally too.

'To stay motivated, I competed against myself. The first time I walked to the station it took me an utterly breathless 45 minutes. After just two weeks, I could do it in 25 minutes. I walked the full 21K half marathon distance in four hours, which was a huge achievement for me, but I'd like to be able to do it in two to three hours one day.

'If I had to pass on what I've learned it would be that anybody can do this plan, regardless of their fitness level or weight. They'll see their fitness levels improve really quickly if they stick at it and believe in themselves.'

Chart your progress

Keep track of your weight loss and fitness success by charting your weekly progress

There's nothing more **motivating than being able to measure the changes in your body shape and fitness as you begin to lose weight and get fitter.** So before you start your 6-week walk-slim plan, I would recommend that you weigh or measure yourself and log your vital statistics.

Then I'd like you to re-measure your stats and weigh-in every week on Mondays – first thing in the morning is best. Stick to this plan and you should really start to notice a big difference in your measurements by week three – if not a little bit sooner – so there will be no excuse to give up!

MEASURE YOUR WEIGHT LOSS

It's not just the scales that tell you how you're shaping up. Muscle weighs more than fat so, to get an idea of how slim and toned you're getting, it's best to measure your vital stats as well as weighing yourself.

Here's what you need to measure:
Bust: measure around the widest part across your nipples.
Waist: take your measurement around your belly button.
Hips: take your measurement around the widest part.
Thigh: measure your right thigh a quarter of the way down from your hip.

MEASURE YOUR FITNESS

As the weight comes off, you'll also be getting fitter. You can measure this by taking your resting heart rate, which should fall as you get fitter. It's a good idea to measure your resting heart rate once a week.

Simply take your pulse, either on your wrist or your neck. Count how many beats there are in 15 seconds then multiply this by four to get your resting heart rate. Make a note of the number and, as you become fitter, you should see this number reduce. That's because your heart becomes more powerful and reduces the amount of beats it produces per minute.

	WEEK 1	WEEK 2	WEEK 3	WEEK 4	WEEK 5	WEEK 6
WEIGHT	106.5	106.5				
BUST ¹¹⁷	124	123				
WAIST	113	108				
HIPS	130	131				
THIGHS	73	77				

RESTING HEART RATE

WEEK 1	68.
WEEK 2	78.
WEEK 3	
WEEK 4	
WEEK 5	
WEEK 6	

do

A good indicator of health and fitness levels is your waist-to-hip ratio (WHR). The ideal ratio is 0.80. Your waist is half way between your hipbone and bottom rib. Measure your hips at the widest point of your bottom and divide your waist measurement by your hips to get the ratio.

CLOTHES: Do Unlimited; dounlimited.com

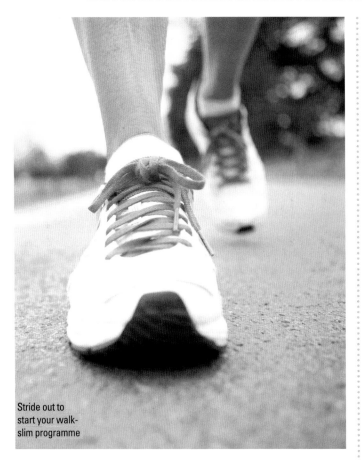

Stride out to start your walk-slim programme

Week: 1

In the first week of the 6-week plan, start gently but stay focused on your goal

At last it's time to start walking yourself slim! Each walking session this week includes bursts of faster walking. These little intervals help burn more fat, increase your fitness and keep your walks interesting. Every week this focus will change. You'll be alternating your walk days with a 4-minute home workout routine (see page 70). This mini workout sounds easy but is quite challenging and will help speed up your metabolism. Again, each week we'll change the focus of the workout. Read on for more details about this week's workouts. And no excuses, let's stick to the plan. If you're motivated by losing weight, try following the diet plan on page 118 this week.

21 *Minute Walk*

THE ROUTINE

▲ **1-minute walk**
Longer stride

▲ **1-minute walk**
Shorter stride

▲ **1-minute walk**
Abdominal pull

Repeat this sequence **7x**

HOW TO DO IT
Longer stride
This will really help to sculpt your hips, legs and bottom. The key is to maintain good upper body posture so that a longer stride is just a slight exaggeration of your normal stride. You should feel your bottom toning with each step.

Shorter stride
Shorten your normal stride very slightly but really focus on using your arms to help power your speed. This gives your arms, obliques and lower body a great workout.

Abdominal pull
Walking at your normal pace, ensuring a good posture, simply pull your belly button tight to your spine and hold for a count of 10 strides then release. Keep repeating for one minute.

WEEK ONE DIARY

Monday: 21-minute walk	*Fill in your progress:* Got to rail bridge. OK!
Tuesday: 4-minute workout: Jogging on the spot fat burner	*Fill in your progress:*
Wednesday: 21-minute walk	*Fill in your progress:* ✓
Thursday: 4-minute workout: Jogging on the spot fat burner	*Fill in your progress:*
Friday: 21-minute walk	*Fill in your progress:* ✓
Saturday: 4-minute workout: Jogging on the spot fat burner	*Fill in your progress:* ✓
Sunday: Rest	*Fill in your progress:*

4-min *workout*

Jogging on the spot fat-burning routine

For this exercise you will need a timer or stop watch, as you have to do it for exactly 4 minutes without stopping.

JOGGING ON THE SPOT

Jog on the spot as fast as you can for **20 seconds.**
Repeat this 8 times.

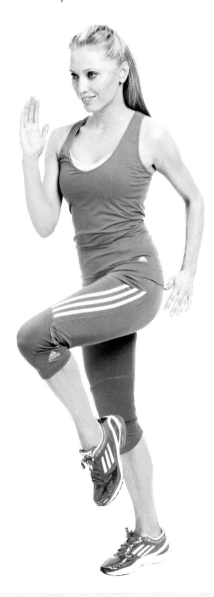

Remember, always to do your warm-up on **page 48**

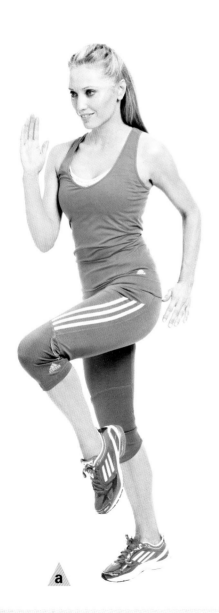

Remember, always do your cool-down stretches on **page 52**

MARCH ON THE SPOT

Then march on the spot for **10 seconds**. **Repeat this 8 times**.

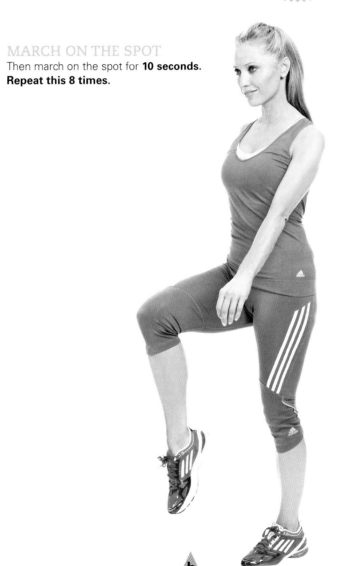

a

b

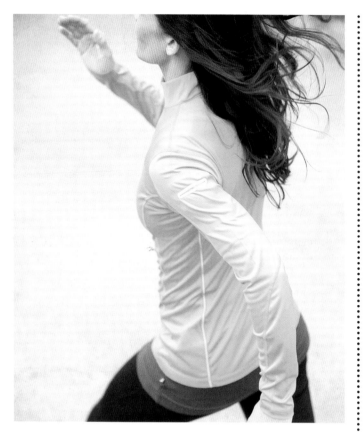

Week: 2

You'll start to notice improvements. Don't slack – even if the weather is bad!

All right girls, it's week 2 of your walk-slim plan. Stick with it and, by the end of next week, you should start to notice a difference. You will find your clothes are starting to feel looser as the inches fall off.

This week we're going to increase the intensity of your walks by doing them for a little longer, as well as giving you a more challenging move for your 4-minute workout.

If you have a day when you're short of time or it's raining and you can't do your walk, then replace it with the 4-minute workout.

Even though 4 minutes sounds easy, it raises the amount of calories you burn. This will vary depending on your age, height and weight but, on average, it can rise by 35 extra calories an hour and can remain high for 10 hours after, so that is 350 calories!

24 *Minute Walk*

THE ROUTINE

▲ **2-minute brisk walk**
Start off with a normal pace, then focus on taking long strides while speeding up to a fast pace.

▲ **1-minute walk**
Shorter Stride
Walk as fast as you can.

▲ **1-minute walk**
Longer Stride
Imagine you're stepping over a puddle. This means you shape and sculpt into your bottom.
Repeat this sequence

6x

HOW TO DO IT
Brisk walk
Start walking at a normal pace then speed up to a brisk pace. Imagine you're walking on a tightrope and place each foot directly in front of the other while swinging your arms naturally.

Longer stride
This will really help to sculpt your hips, legs and bottom. The key is to maintain good upper body posture so that a longer stride is just a slight exaggeration of your normal stride. You should feel your bottom toning with each step.

Shorter stride
Shorten your normal stride very slightly but really focus on using your arms here to help power your speed. This gives your arms, obliques and lower body a great workout.

WEEK TWO DIARY

Monday: 24-minute walk	*Fill in your progress:*	Felt the extra bit!
Tuesday: 4-minute workout: Inner and outer thigh sculptor	*Fill in your progress:*	
Wednesday: 24-minute walk	*Fill in your progress:*	
Thursday: 4-minute workout: Inner and outer thigh sculptor	*Fill in your progress:*	
Friday: 24-minute walk	*Fill in your progress:*	
Saturday: 4-minute workout: Inner and outer thigh sculptor	*Fill in your progress:*	
Sunday: Rest	*Fill in your progress:*	

4-min workout

Inner and outer thigh sculptor routine

You'll need a timer or stop watch for this exercise, as you have to do it for exactly **4 minutes** without stopping.

JUMP UP

Jump up high so you create a star shape. Repeat as fast as you can for **20 seconds. Pause then repeat this 8 times.**

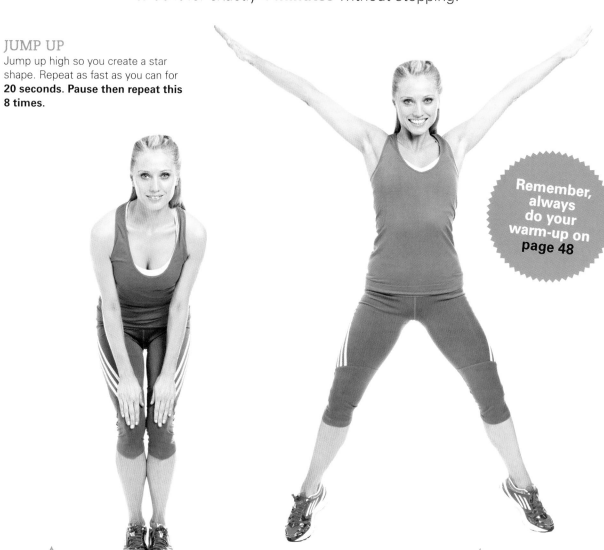

Remember, always do your warm-up on **page 48**

a

b

Remember, always do your cool-down stretches on **page 52**

MARCH ON THE SPOT

Then march on the spot for **10 seconds.**
Repeat this 8 times.

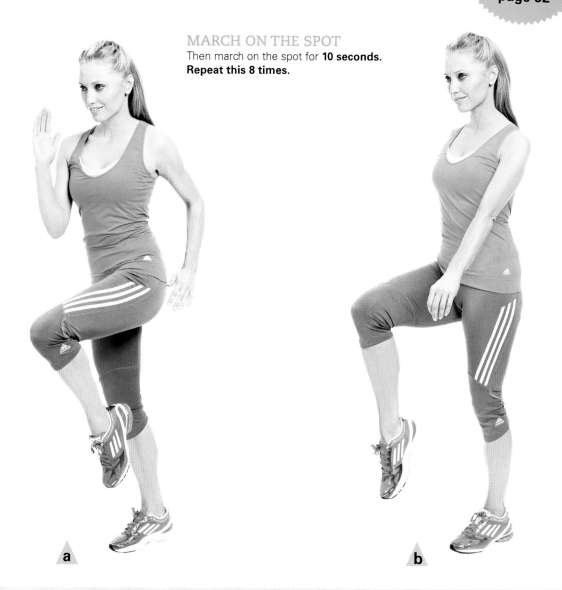

a

b

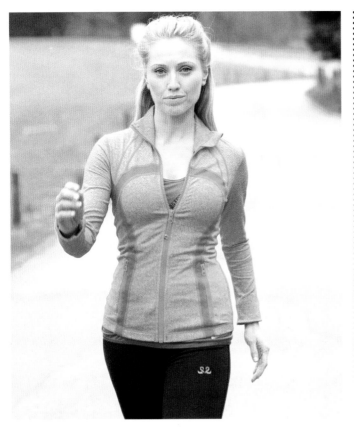

Week: 3

You'll be feeling fitter and more toned, and able to cope with longer walks this week

f you have managed to stay on track with your workouts and eating plan then, by the end of this week, you should notice a real difference in your body shape and fitness. And you may even be going down a dress size, too.

This week we are going to increase the intensity of your walks by doing them for a little longer but don't worry, they'll still be easy to squeeze into your lunch hour. We'll be working on giving you killer curves with a great waist-toning exercise.

For your 4-minute workout, this week we're going to focus on a low-impact exercise – but don't be fooled, it is still really tough. This workout is great for not only burning up those calories but also for toning your waist and arms so you'll look good in summer tops and T-shirts.

30 *Minute Walk*

THE ROUTINE

▲ **2-minute brisk walk**
Start off with a good pace, then focus on taking long strides while keeping up a fast pace.

▲ **1-minute super-fast walk**
Walk as fast as you can, keeping your stride small and pump through with your arms. Be sure not to lock out your knee joints.

Repeat this sequence

HOW TO DO IT
Brisk walk
Start walking at a normal pace then speed up to a brisk pace. Imagine you're walking on a tightrope and place each foot directly in front of the other while swinging your arms naturally.

Longer stride
This will really help to sculpt your hips, legs and bottom. The key is to maintain good upper body posture so that a longer stride is just a slight exaggeration of your normal stride. You should feel your bottom toning with each step.

Shorter stride
Shorten your normal stride very slightly but really focus on using your arms here to help power your speed. This gives your arms, obliques and lower body a great workout.

WEEK THREE DIARY

Monday: 30-minute walk	*Fill in your progress:*
Tuesday: 4-minute workout: Waist and arm toner	*Fill in your progress:*
Wednesday: 30-minute walk	*Fill in your progress:*
Thursday: 4-minute workout: Waist and arm toner	*Fill in your progress:*
Friday: 30-minute walk	*Fill in your progress:*
Saturday: 4-minute workout: Waist and arm toner	*Fill in your progress:*
Sunday: Rest	*Fill in your progress:*

4-min workout

Waist and arm toner routine

For this exercise you'll need a timer or stop watch, as you have to do it for exactly **4 minutes** without stopping.

ARM PUNCH

To do this, stand in a wide stance with your knees bent. Punch your arms back and forth as fast as you can without twisting your hips for **20 seconds.** To work harder, punch your arms higher. **Repeat this 8 times.**

Remember, always do your warm-up on **page 48**

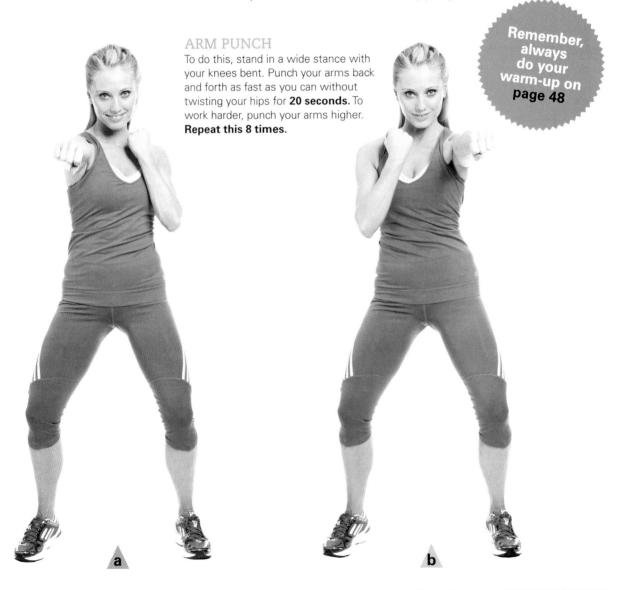

a

b

Remember, always to do your cool-down stretches on **page 52**

MARCH ON THE SPOT
Then march on the spot for **10 seconds**.
Repeat this 8 times.

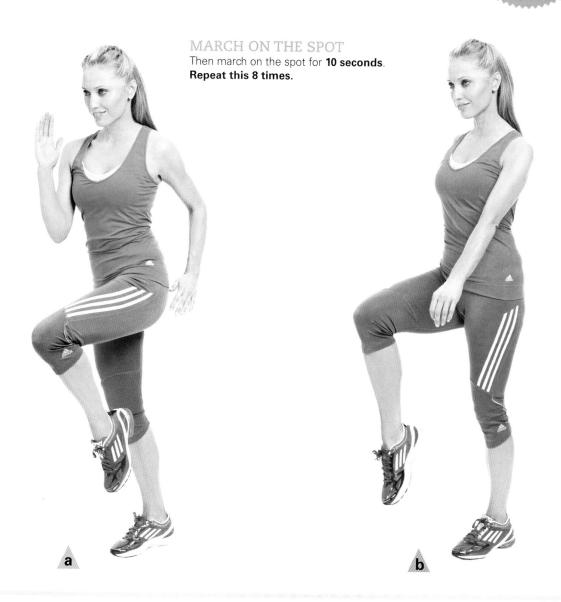

a

b

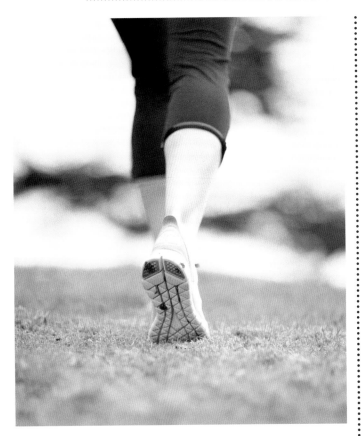

Week: 4

The walks are shorter this week but the workout is challenging – it will be worth it!

You're half way through the 6-week plan now and **you'll be looking amazing and feeling super fit if you can stick it out this week.** There's no time for relaxing – we are now going to up the intensity again. We're going to shorten your walks by five minutes but make the intervals much more of a challenge!

For your 4-minute workout, this week we are going to do a more challenging sequence called the lower body power workout, which involves jumping from side to side. It helps if you have a yoga block, a book or even a cushion to jump over. If you do find this workout too strenuous, simply step rather than jump and then do a squat. This will help to define and sculpt your legs and bottom.

25 *Minute Walk*

THE ROUTINE

▲ 1-minute brisk walk
Focus on taking long strides while keeping up a fast pace.

▲ 1-minute crossed arms walk
Walk at a good fast pace, but have your arms crossed over your chest. This means all the work comes from your hips and you feel it working on your abs, hips and bottom.

▲ 3-minute super-fast walk
Walk as fast as you can keeping your stride small and pump through with your arms. Be sure not to lock your knee joints.

Repeat this sequence

5x

HOW TO DO IT

Longer stride
This will help to sculpt through your hips, legs and bottom. The key is to maintain good upper body posture so that a longer stride is a slight exaggeration of your normal stride and you feel your bottom toning with each step.

Crossed arms walk
Crossing your arms means they can't help propel you forwards, so your abs, hips and bottom have to work harder.

Shorter stride
Shorten your normal stride very slightly but really focus on using your arms here to help power your speed. This gives your arms, obliques and lower body a great workout.

WEEK FOUR DIARY

Monday:
25-minute walk

Fill in your progress:

Tuesday:
4-minute workout:
Lower body power workout

Fill in your progress:

Wednesday:
25-minute walk

Fill in your progress:

Thursday:
4-minute workout:
Lower body power workout

Fill in your progress:

Friday:
25-minute walk

Fill in your progress:

Saturday:
4-minute workout:
Lower body power workout

Fill in your progress:

Sunday:
Rest

Fill in your progress:

4-min workout

Lower-body power workout

For this exercise you will need a timer or stop watch, as you have to do this for exactly **4 minutes** without stopping. You'll also need a cushion, yoga block or book.

SQUAT JUMPS

Stand in a narrow stance with your knees bent. Place a yoga block on the floor to your side. Jump over it from side to side. If this is too tough, just step over it. Do it for **20 seconds. Repeat this 8 times.**

Remember, always do your warm-up on **page 48**

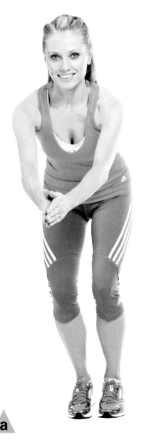

a

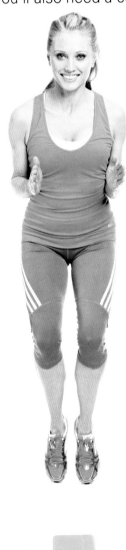

b

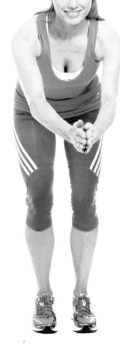

c

Remember, always do your cool-down stretches on **page 52**

MARCH ON THE SPOT

March on the spot for **10 seconds.**
Repeat this 8 times.

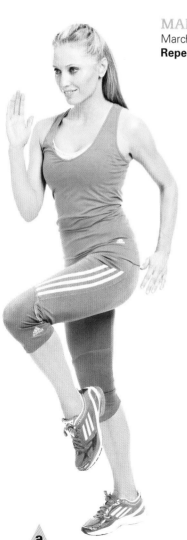

a

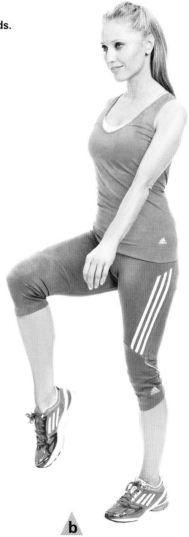

b

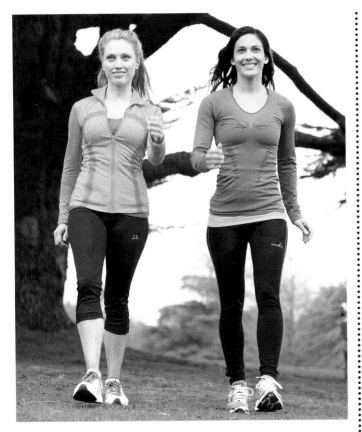

Week: 5

The pounds are falling off and you're feeling fit – the plan is really working

By now you should really be noticing that your clothes are looser as the inches and pounds drop off. But, just as importantly, you should be feeling so much fitter with increased energy levels – and you may even find that you're sleeping a lot better.

So, again, I'm going to crank up the intensity this week. You should be able to cope with it as you'll be feeling so much fitter than you did at the beginning of the plan. I'm knocking a minute off your walks and making you work hard at your intervals.

This week, your 4-minute workout is a really challenging mountain climber exercise. These strenuous floor-based moves are a fantastic calorie burner and will give your abs, arms and legs a great toning workout as well.

24 *Minute Walk*

THE ROUTINE

▲ **1-minute brisk walk**

▲ **1-minute crossed arms walk**
This gives your abs, hips and bottom a great workout.

▲ **3-minute super-fast walk**
Walk at your fastest pace using a short stride and pump through with your arms. Don't lock your knee joints.

▲ **1-minute walk**
Abdominal pull

Repeat this sequence

4x

HOW TO DO IT

Longer stride
The key is to maintain good upper body posture so a longer stride is a slight exaggeration of your normal stride and you feel your bottom toning as you walk.

Crossed arms walk
Crossing your arms means they can't help propel you forwards so your abs, hips and bottom have to work harder.

Shorter stride
This is shortening your normal stride a little while using your arms to help power your speed. It gives your arms, obliques and lower body a great workout.

Abdominal pull
Walking at a brisk pace, pull your belly button tight to your spine and hold for a count of 10 strides then release and keep repeating throughout the minute.

WEEK FIVE DIARY

Monday: 24-minute walk	*Fill in your progress:*
Tuesday: 4-minute workout: Mountain climber workout	*Fill in your progress:*
Wednesday: 24-minute walk	*Fill in your progress:*
Thursday: 4-minute workout: Mountain climber workout	*Fill in your progress:*
Friday: 24-minute walk	*Fill in your progress:*
Saturday: 4-minute workout: Mountain climber workout	*Fill in your progress:*
Sunday: Rest	*Fill in your progress:*

4-min *workout*

Mountain climber routine

For this exercise you will need a timer or stop watch, as you have to do it for exactly **4 minutes** without stopping.

Remember, always do your warm-up on **page 48**

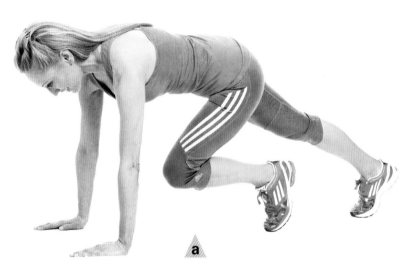

a

CLIMBING ROUTINE

Come onto the floor on your hands and feet and bring your left knee into your chest. Then swap your legs as if you're performing a running movement, while keeping your tummy pulled in. If you find this too hard – it is very challenging – just bring your legs in slower.
Do this for 20 seconds.
Repeat 8 times.

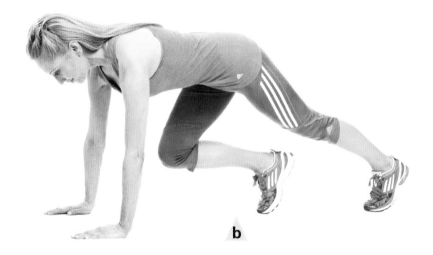

b

RESTING POSE

Kneel on your hands and knees for **10 seconds.** Slowly come up into a standing position. **Repeat 8 times.**

Remember, always do your cool-down stretches on **page 52**

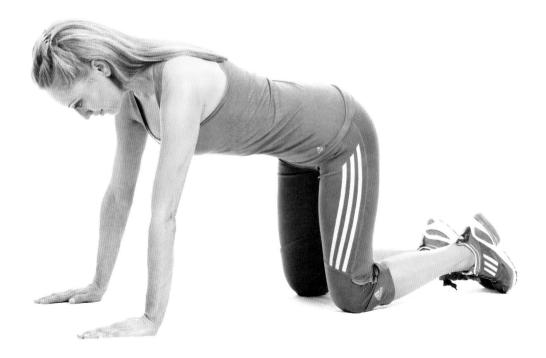

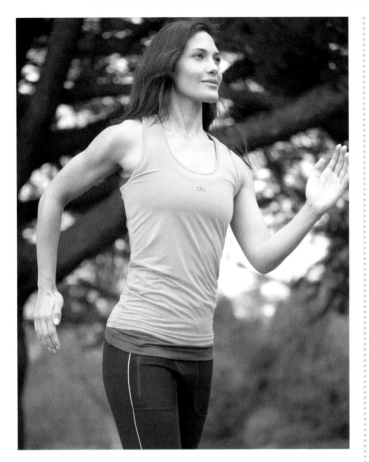

Week: 6

Well done! You've reached the final week and you should be proud of the new you

You have now arrived at your final week of the walk-slim plan and you should be feeling fabulous – all trim and fit and bursting with energy. But let's give it a real push and go for gold on this last week so that we can make sure you've achieved all the fitness and weight-loss goals you set yourself at the beginning.

This last week consists of the usual interval walking, along with your 4-minute challenge, which is jumping lunges again. This is a very tough exercise but it does get results. If you find it too difficult, you can always take out the jump to make the workout a little less challenging.

30 *Minute Walk*

THE ROUTINE

▲ **1-minute walk**
Longer stride
Pull your tummy muscles in tight.

▲ **1-minute walk**
Shorter stride
Go faster and pump with your arms.

▲ **1-minute crossed arms walk**
Walk as fast as you can with arms crossed on your chest. This works your abs, hips and bottom.

▲ **1-minute walk**
Abdominal pull

Repeat this sequence **6x**

HOW TO DO IT

Longer stride
The key is to maintain good upper body posture so a longer stride is a slight exaggeration of your normal stride and you feel your bottom toning as you walk.

Crossed arms walk
Crossing your arms means they can't help propel you forwards so your abs, hips and bottom have to work harder.

Shorter stride
Shorten your normal stride while using your arms to help power your speed. It gives your arms, obliques and lower body a great workout.

Abdominal pull
Walking at a brisk pace, ensuring good posture, pull your belly button tight to your spine and hold for a count of 10 strides. Release and repeat.

WEEK SIX DIARY

Monday: 30-minute walk	*Fill in your progress:*
Tuesday: 4-minute workout: Jumping lunges	*Fill in your progress:*
Wednesday: 30-minute walk	*Fill in your progress:*
Thursday: 4-minute workout: Jumping lunges	*Fill in your progress:*
Friday: 30-minute walk	*Fill in your progress:*
Saturday: 4-minute workout: Jumping lunges	*Fill in your progress:*
Sunday: Rest	*Fill in your progress:*

4-min *workout*

Jumping lunges routine

You'll need a timer or stop watch for this exercise, as you have to do it for exactly 4 minutes without stopping.

JUMPING LUNGES

Stand with your left knee bent at a 90° angle, your right leg behind you and your arms in front **(a)**. Jump **(b)** and land with your right knee bent and left leg behind **(c)**. Do it for **20 seconds**. **Repeat this 8 times.**

Remember, always do your warm-up on **page 48**

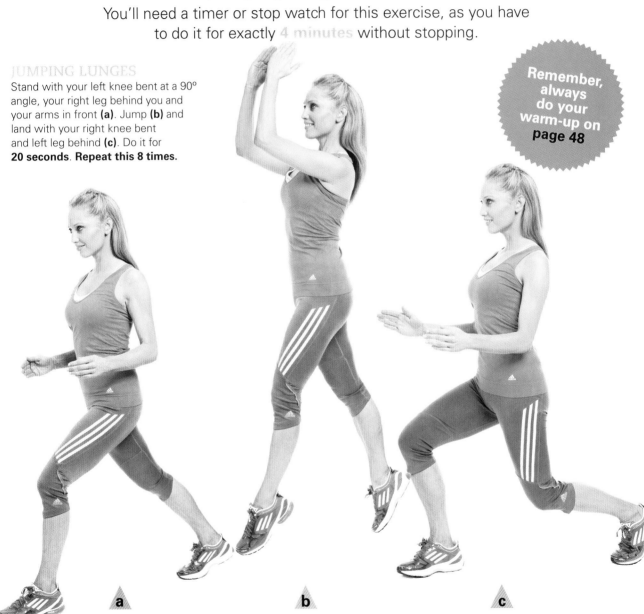

a   b   c

Remember,
always
do your
cool-down
stretches on
page 52

MARCH ON THE SPOT

Then march on the spot for **10 seconds.**
Shake out your arms for a quick rest then
go again. **Repeat this 8 times.**

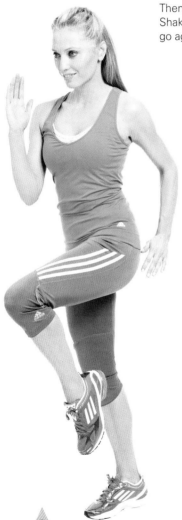

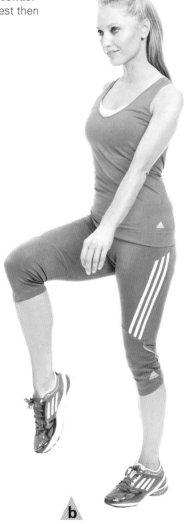

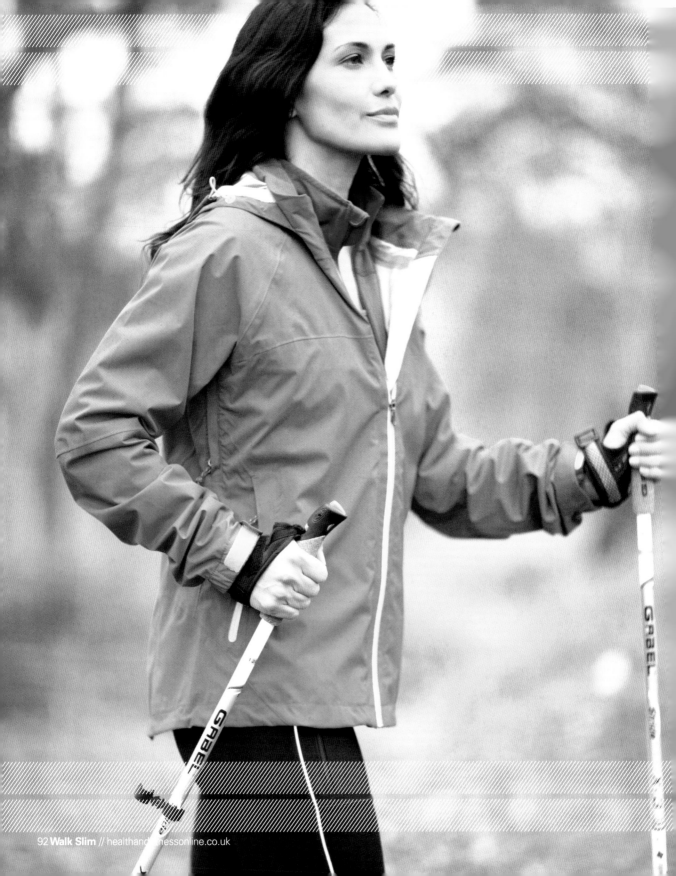

WALK ON

Congratulations, you've completed the 6-week walk-slim plan and should be feeling and looking amazing. You can feel proud of what you've achieved. So don't stop! Now you're in the walking habit, it's the perfect time to make power walking a permanent part of your daily life. This chapter is packed with ideas to help you do this – from becoming an active commuter and setting up a walking group to entering a race.
Read on to start reaping the rewards today!

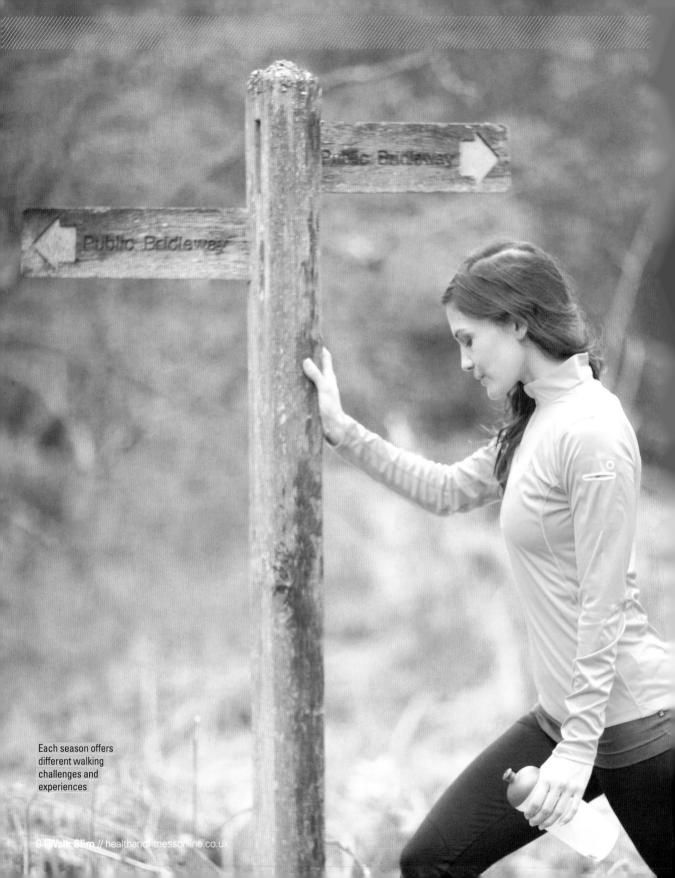

Public Bridleway

Public Bridleway

Each season offers
different walking
challenges and
experiences

Taking it further

Now you've got the walking habit, it's time to add some new challenges

As walking's now part of your lifestyle, it's the perfect time to find new ways to keep it fresh, exciting and challenging. Finding ways to incorporate more walking into your daily life, and to make each walk more varied and challenging, will ensure you maintain and increase the body benefits you've already started to enjoy.

One great way to stay on track is to sign up for some walking events. These days, many charity races are open to walkers as well as runners, from 5K and 10K events to full marathons. There are more popping up all over the country. See page 108 for a list of events to enter.

Turn your walks into a social event by getting friends or family together and planning some spring, summer, winter and autumn walks. Browse online for inspiration on locations and routes. Book in some dates and plan to make a day of it. Each season offers different challenges and experiences depending on the weather and countryside. If you enjoy the social aspect of walking, think about setting up a regular walking date with friends. See page 104 for advice on how to set up a walking group.

Whenever you can, think walk not drive. Most of us jump in our cars as it's quick and easy but if you have a short drive to do a quick errand, get into the habit of ditching the car keys and putting on your trainers instead. Turn to page 97 to find out more about how to become an active commuter. Incorporate power walking into your day to get fit without needing the gym!

5 REASONS TO WALK NOT DRIVE!

DRIVING
- Sitting down while driving doesn't tone or sculpt your body.
- Stress of parking or traffic jams.
- Costs money in fuel and parking.
- Puts mileage on your car.
- Bad for the planet.

WALKING
- Brisk walking helps shape and tone you.
- Feel-good factor – walking helps release endorphins, the feel-good hormones.
- Saves money – no fuel and no parking tickets.
- The more you walk, the more calories you burn.
- Good for the planet.

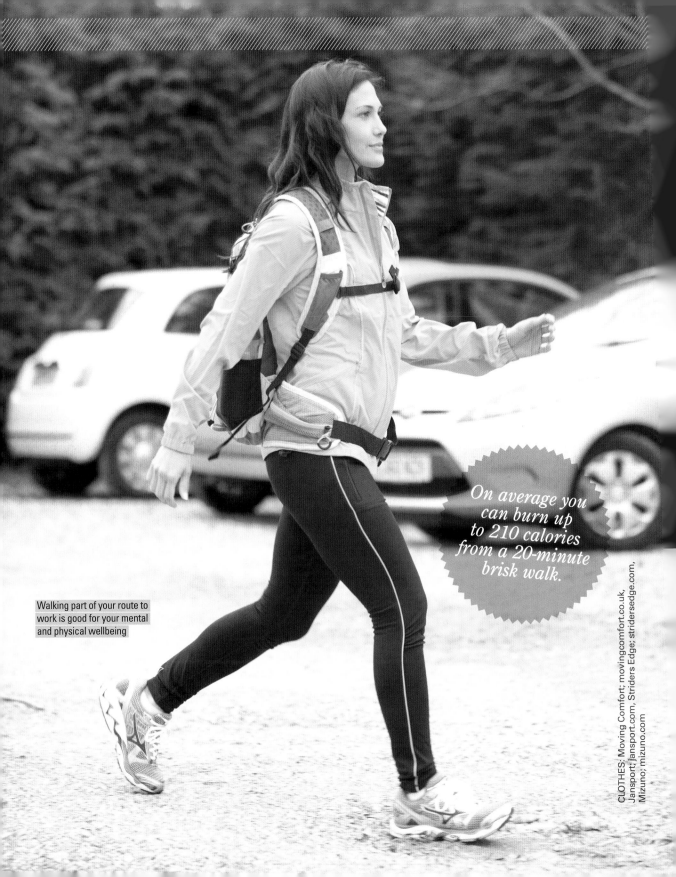

On average you can burn up to 210 calories from a 20-minute brisk walk.

Walking part of your route to work is good for your mental and physical wellbeing

Walk to work

Get fit on your way to and from the office by becoming an active commuter

Your commute to and from work is the ideal time to add some walking into your daily life. It's a great way to clear your thoughts, de-stress, re-energise – and save money. Even if you can't walk the whole of your journey, you can find ways to change the route so that you only drive or take the bus half way and walk the rest.

If you commute into the city by train, try taking a break from the tube and walk to work from your mainline station. A couple of active commutes a week can make a big difference to your size and weight. On average, you can burn up to 210 calories from a 20-minute brisk walk. Do this four times a week and that's an extra 840 calories you'll burn off, plus money saved from your regular commute.

And you'll feel more energised than if you were stuck in a stressful traffic jam or crammed into the tube! Try taking the stairs rather than lifts or escalators, to tone up your bottom and boost your calorie burn throughout the day.

MAP YOUR ROUTE

Keep your active commute interesting by exploring different routes. It's a great way to get to know your town or city and discover or rediscover some of the sights you've taken for granted for years. There are plenty of on-line tools to help you find and plan routes.

● **walkit.com**
This site can help you plan a route in more than 29 UK cities, including information on the possible journey time, calorie burn, step count and

> ❝❝ WALK TO WORK FROM THE STATION. A FEW ACTIVE COMMUTES A WEEK CAN MAKE A DIFFERENCE TO YOUR SIZE AND WEIGHT ❝❝

how much carbon you've saved. The site now includes circular route planning – perfect for lunchtime walks with your workmates.

● **tfl.gov.uk/gettingaround/walking**
If you live in London, Transport for London's Journey Planner has walking options. Use the link to select the Walking Journey Planner. If you aren't interested in using any other modes of transport on your journey, make sure you deselect those boxes. This link has lists of strategic walking routes in London. TFL also has a host of other tools to help you get around – it's well worth a look. 〉〉〉〉

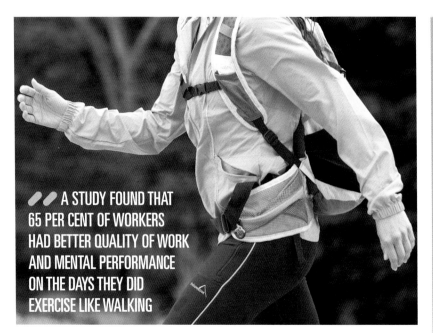

A STUDY FOUND THAT 65 PER CENT OF WORKERS HAD BETTER QUALITY OF WORK AND MENTAL PERFORMANCE ON THE DAYS THEY DID EXERCISE LIKE WALKING

WALK AT WORK

Why not get your colleagues walking too, to boost your motivation and help others get healthy? Ask your managers to start promoting walking at work. A study at Leeds Metropolitan University, found that 65 per cent of workers had better quality of work, mental performance and time management on the days when they did exercise such as walking. Every May, pedestrian's charity Living Streets organises an event called Walk to Work Week to get the nation walking. Here are some ideas to help promote it in your workplace.

1 The pedometer test
It's hard to know if you're walking enough each day. Ask your managers to issue a pedometer to each employee. They're a great way to get people thinking about how much they really walk.

2 Sticker your lift
Sometimes taking the lift is far too tempting, so post messages on and around your company lifts to encourage fellow workers to walk.

3 Company reminder
Choose a regular date once a week or once a month encouraging everyone to walk at least 15 minutes on their way to work. Set this up in all staff calendars with a reminder going out the day before.

4 Don't email it, walk it
Ban internal emails one day a week and see how much more walking employees do.

5 Mobile meetings
Who said you had to sit down for a meeting? Try to set up walking meetings to get those ideas flowing.

6 Lunch hour walks
Make the most of lunch breaks by combining walking and socialising with a 'walk at lunch time' group.

7 Sign up your work place for Walk to Work Week
At livingstreets.org.uk you'll be able to log how many miles everyone walked, calories burnt and carbon footprint savings.

WHAT YOU NEED CONTINUED...

SMART SHOES
These MBT trainers will activate your muscles while you walk – and stand still. They encourage greater muscle activity, reduce lower back pain and improve posture. **MBT Mahuta Shoes, £179.99; johnlewis.com**

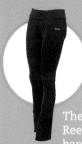

FITNESS TROUSERS
Try wearing toning fitness bottoms to add extra oomph to your walk. These ones have Reebok ResisTone bands sewn into the design to work your muscles harder with every step. They also give your lower back extra support. **Reebok EasyTone Pant, £55; reebok.com**

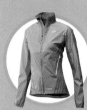

JACKET
Stash a bright, waterproof jacket in your backpack if you need to remove a layer. It's ideal for all weathers as the soft shell combines protection with breathable material. A hood will protect you from unexpected downpours and stretch fabric is extra comfortable. **Adidas Terrex Hybrid Softshell Jacket, £125; adidas.com**

Make walking part of your workout

www.livingstreets.org.uk/fitness

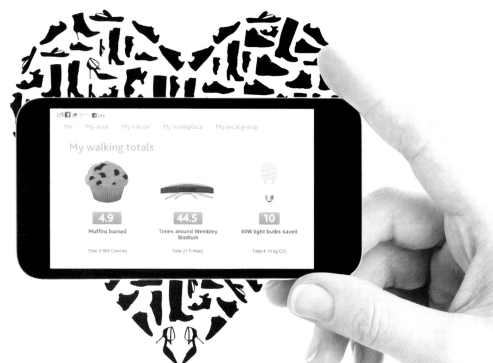

Sign up to My Living Streets to create your FREE online walking log:

- Track miles walked, calories burned and CO_2 saved
- Take part in challenges to earn rewards
- Get involved in campaigns to improve your streets.

Start logging your miles at
www.livingstreets.org.uk/fitness

LIVING STREETS
PUTTING PEOPLE FIRST

Company Registration No. 5368409 Registered Charity No. 1108448 (England and Wales) and SC039808 (Scotland)

Indoor training

Handy and weatherproof, taking your walks indoors has benefits

While nothing beats walking outdoors, jumping on a treadmill – whether at home or at the gym – can be a convenient way to up your walking quota. While outdoor walking offers the benefits of fresh air and inspiring views, treadmills have advantages too. You can monitor your distance walked and calories burned plus you have access to hill climbs, all at the touch of a button.

The gym is also a lot safer than dark streets for solo walkers and is less stressful on the body than concrete, so it's a good option if you're injury prone. However, without environmental factors, such as wind and uneven terrain, and with the conveyer-like 'pulling' effect on your feet, treadmills can make walking less challenging. Here's how to get the most out of your indoor walking workouts.

GET MORE FROM THE TREADMILL

1 For a smooth stride, take slightly longer steps than usual, since the belt is pulling your foot back. To avoid hunching on an incline, lean forward from your ankles. And remember not to bend at your waist.

> THE GYM IS A LOT SAFER THAN DARK STREETS FOR SOLO WALKERS, AND LESS STRESSFUL ON THE BODY THAN CONCRETE

2 Try setting the incline to at least one per cent to match the demands of the outdoors. Research from Brighton University shows that having the belt on a slight incline compensates for the lack of wind resistance and varied terrain that would make walking in the 'real world' more challenging.

YOUR TREADMILL WARM-UP

Ease yourself into your workout and warm up your muscles by walking at 2mph for one minute, then walk on your toes at 1.5mph for 30 seconds, and then 30 seconds on your heels. Set an incline of five and take longer strides for one minute. Finally, return the incline setting to 0 and walk for two minutes at 3-3.5mph.

3 Avoid looking down at the belt or machine controls. Stand tall, with your eyes gazing straight ahead. Use the mirrors to assess your walking posture and technique.

4 Don't just plod along at the same old speed. Make the most of the machine's features, such as pre-set sessions, hills and varied pace, to add variety to your workout. Or create your own interval sessions, using the distance or time buttons. Why not race a friend for extra motivation and added interest?

5 Enter your age and weight correctly, so you get accurate readings for calorie burn and heart rate. Ask your gym if you can borrow a chest strap, so that the heart-rate measurements are precise.

6 Listen to your favourite motivating music to power your walking and help beat boredom.

7 Listen to your feet. If you hear a loud thumping, you're landing flat-footed. Try landing on your heel and rolling through the ball of your foot to your toes.

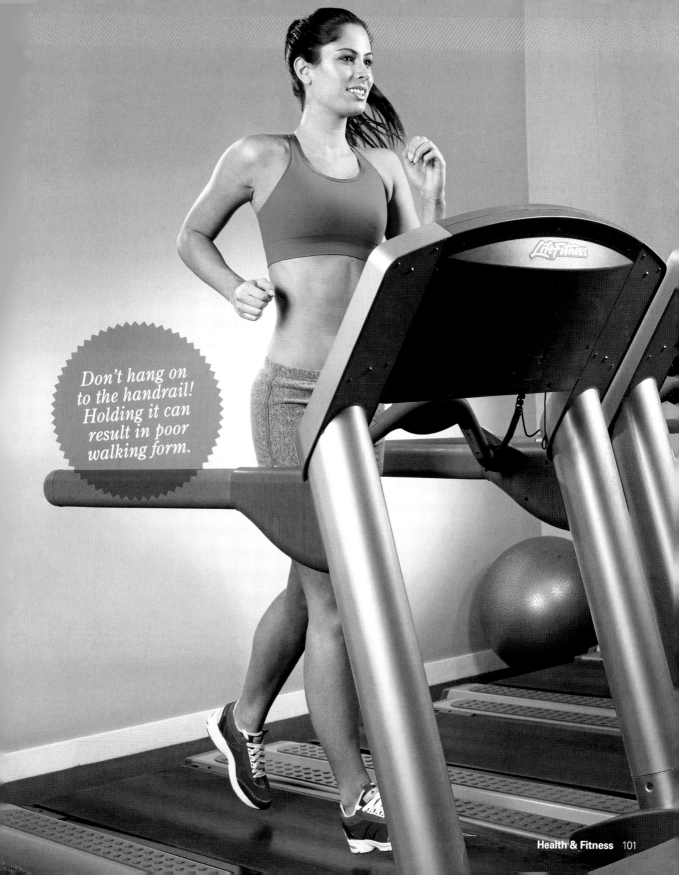

Don't hang on to the handrail! Holding it can result in poor walking form.

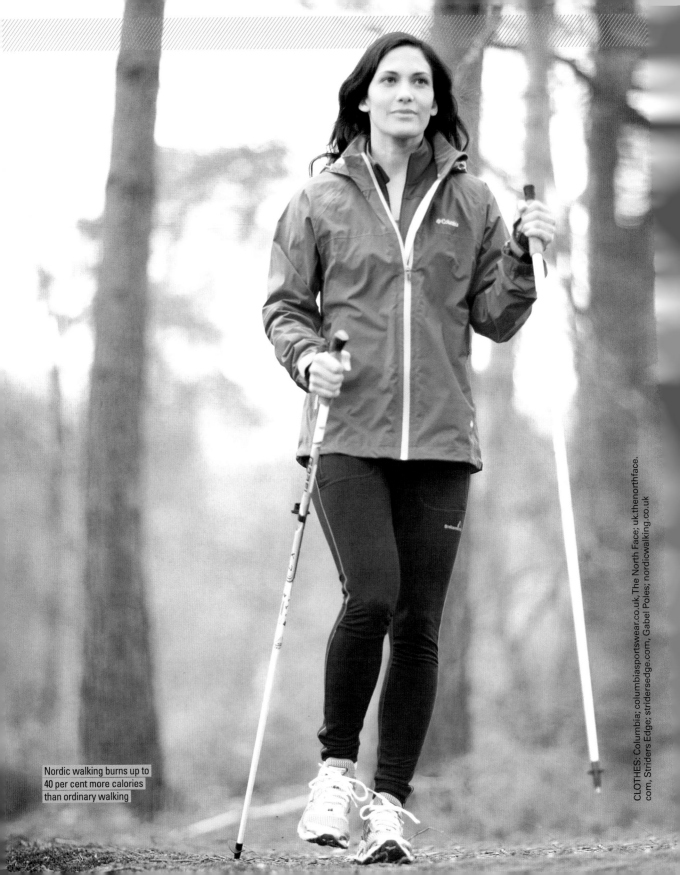

Nordic walking burns up to 40 per cent more calories than ordinary walking

CLOTHES: Columbia; columbiasportswear.co.uk, The North Face; uk.thenorthface.com, Striders Edge; stridersedge.com, Gabel Poles; nordicwalking.co.uk

Nordic walking

Burn more calories and tone your upper body by adding a pair of poles into the mix

f you've seen people walking in the countryside with a pair of long poles, they're not techno geeks, they're Nordic walking. Originally a way for cross-country skiiers to have a workout during the summer, these super-long walking poles are designed to harness the power of your upper body to help propel you forwards. It's a great way to turn an ordinary walk into a whole-body workout – a bit like using a cross-trainer, only you're outdoors.

The great thing about Nordic walking is it's suitable for everyone, no matter what your age or fitness level. Not only will it strengthen your major muscle groups, using poles also takes the pressure off your joints, making it ideal if you're new to exercise, recovering from an injury or want a low-impact way to boost your fitness. In fact, Nordic walking provides the same aerobic benefits as running or swimming, but feels easier because the poles aid your movement.

You'll also burn up to 40 per cent more calories than with ordinary walking, and, as your technique improves, your muscles become more metabolically active – meaning you'll burn even more calories. Studies have shown the technique alleviates neck and shoulder pain, increases hip-bone density and reduces depression and fatigue, compared with control groups who walked without poles.

GET KITTED OUT

To get started, all you need is a pair of Nordic walking poles and flexible outdoor shoes or trainers. Most instructors will provide equipment, but you can buy poles for about £30 (try nordicwalking.co.uk/store). If you're a

> **IT'S A GREAT WAY TO TURN AN ORDINARY WALK INTO A WHOLE-BODY EXERCISE – LIKE USING A CROSSTRAINER ONLY OUTDOORS**

beginner, choose poles with a variable length. That way you can adjust them according to the terrain you're walking on. Once you're more experienced you can lengthen or shorten them as you settle into the rhythm that suits you.

HOW TO DO IT

The best way to learn is with a qualified instructor. You'll need about four sessions to learn the correct technique to engage the right muscles to enable you to get maximum benefits. If you want to try it yourself, focus on the following:

● With one pole in each hand, start walking normally, letting your arms swing freely from your shoulders with your elbows straight. Walk and drag the poles behind you. The poles attach to your hands via wrist straps, so you don't need to grip them too tightly.
● Gradually, push through from your shoulder, planting the poles more firmly into the ground.
● Once you've mastered the basic technique, you can try more advanced moves that add resistance and boost your heart rate, such as double poling and Nordic striding. These are best learned with an instructor who will build up the technique in 'layers' to make sure you're using the correct muscles. You'll be amazed how much faster and further you can walk.

GIVE IT A GO

There are more than 2,000 qualified instructors throughout the UK. To find your nearest, log on to **nordicwalking.co.uk**, go to 'Find a Class' and enter your postcode. For your FREE taster, tick the box to show instructors taking part in promotions.

Set up a walking group

Have fun while you get fit by turning your walks into a social occasion

PRAM POWER

If you want to lose your baby weight and it's at least six weeks after the birth (or 10 weeks following a C-section), it's safe to start exercising again. Walking is a safe way to shape up, lose belly fat and retone your pelvic floor muscles. The latest post-natal exercise craze is for power pramming – exercising outdoors while pushing your baby in its pram. Companies such as Pushy Mothers (pushymothers.com), Buggy Fit (buggyfit.co.uk) and Powerpramming (powerpramming. co.uk) hold classes across London and the UK. They're taught by approved post-natal instructors and there are stops for core stability, strength and stretching exercises. The fresh air and company boosts your mood and staves off any post-baby blues.

Get back in shape after giving birth with power pramming

Walking is the perfect social exercise. Inviting friends or family to walk with you is a great way to make your walks more fun and enjoyable – and it should ensure you stick to your plan!

Why not think about creating your own walking group? Simply find several people who are keen to get or stay fit and stay slim, and set a day and time that suits you all. Book a regular date in the diary – once you're committed to meeting up you'll be less likely to cancel. Not only is walking in a group often more motivating, it's also safer, especially on those darker evenings during the winter.

MEET YOUR FRIENDS

Decide on a weekly meeting spot or perhaps take it in turns to set the routes or pace. You could do a round circuit, or see if you can increase your time or distance each week. For a weekend treat, choose a route that ends at a pub for a lovely lazy lunch.

Why not create your own walk-slim page on Facebook? Invite your friends to join you and update each other on your progress and chat about your weekly walks. It's free to set up and is a great way to keep in touch with your friends and motivate each other to get fit.

WORK OUT AT WORK

Alternatively, organise a walk-slim group at your workplace and hold 20-30 minute walks on alternate days, for instance Mondays, Wednesdays and Fridays. Not only will your boss be impressed at how energised and productive you are on your return, compared with those who've lounged around eating lunch at their desks – you'll notice the difference too!

If you're a new mum, walking is the perfect way to work off that baby weight. So how about getting a group of mum friends together for walks? Use the time while your children are at nursery or school – or take your children with you in their buggies!

Power pramming (see panel, left) is a popular new way for women with children to exercise but you don't have to join a class, you can easily organise your own pram walks.

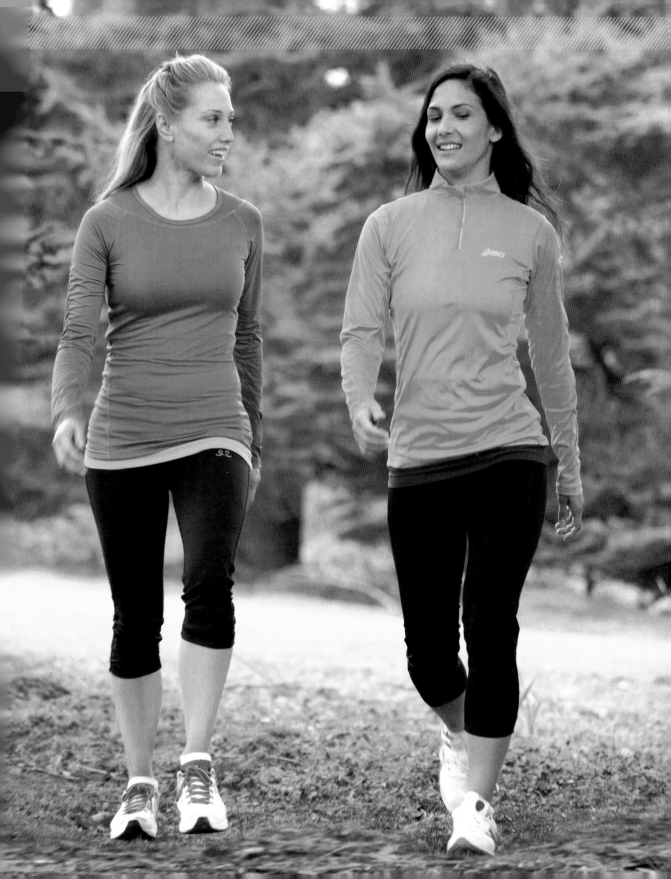

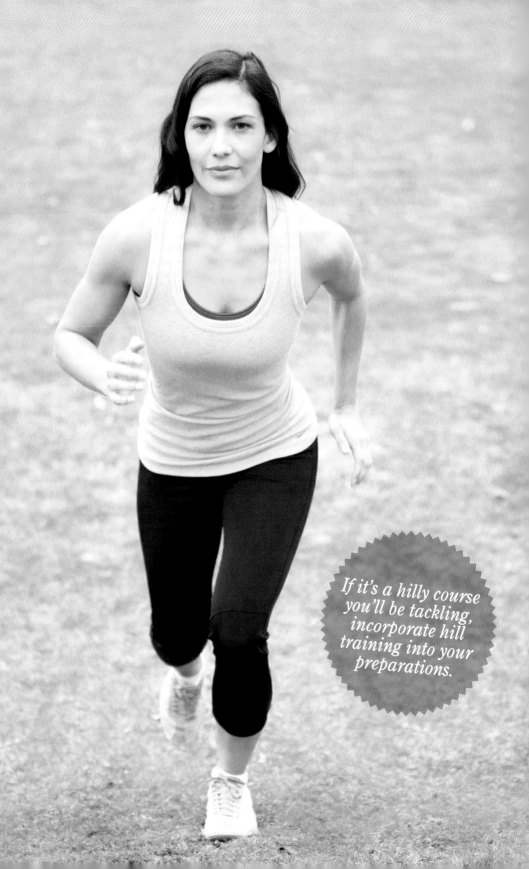

If it's a hilly course you'll be tackling, incorporate hill training into your preparations.

Signing up for a charity challenge can motivate you to keep walking

Charity challenge

Add purpose to your walking programme by pledging to raise money for a good cause while you get fit

Charity walks are the perfect way to help you reach your fitness goals and give you a feel-good factor. What better motivation to stick to your training programme than knowing you'll be helping others as you get fitter? These days, there's a huge variety of charity walks to choose from, ranging from the Cancer Research 5K Race for Life events, held across the UK every summer (raceforlife.org) to the Moonwalk marathon (walkthewalk. org) held in London and Edinburgh.

To find the right event for you, be realistic about your fitness levels and decide how long you want to walk for – are you more suited to a short but fast-paced event, or a longer endurance challenge? Seek out an event that will stretch you and encourage you to up your training, but isn't so extreme that you'll drop out beforehand or fail to complete the event on the big day.

HOW TO TRAIN
Whatever the distance of your charity walk, it's vital to train properly. The more training you do and the more miles you cover, the more enjoyment and success you'll have on the day, so make sure you give yourself sufficient time to train.

If you're a beginner, you can train for a 5K walk in five to eight weeks, doing three to four walks a week. If you're already walking regularly, you can take on something more challenging. It's possible to train for a half-marathon walk in 12 weeks and a full marathon

> ❞❞ BE REALISTIC ABOUT YOUR FITNESS LEVELS AND DECIDE HOW LONG YOU WANT TO WALK FOR ❞❞

in 16 weeks. For more advice and training tips, visit walkthewalk.org. Try to cover similar terrain to that you'll be walking during the event, especially if it's a hilly course.

As well as doing progressively longer walking sessions, try to cross-train with other activities such as swimming or yoga to help build your strength and flexibility and rest your walking muscles. Include one or two rest days a week to give your muscles a chance to recover. On these days, try to do a 10-minute stretch session to keep your muscles flexible and prevent injury. You could even do these while you're watching TV, just make sure you're nice and warm before you start. Aim to do at least one walk of a similar distance to your event, two to three weeks beforehand, so you know what to expect on the day. This is the ideal time to test any kit or snacks you'll be using, and if it's a hilly course, use hill training in your preparations.

You also need to prepare yourself mentally for the challenge. You might feel nervous beforehand – if so, it could help to write down your concerns. Then, think of strategies to overcome them, such as enlisting the support of friends and family to help you stick to your training plan, or asking them not to offer you unhealthy snacks. Planning your route to the venue and packing your bag in advance will all help you feel more in control and leave you free to enjoy yourself on the day.

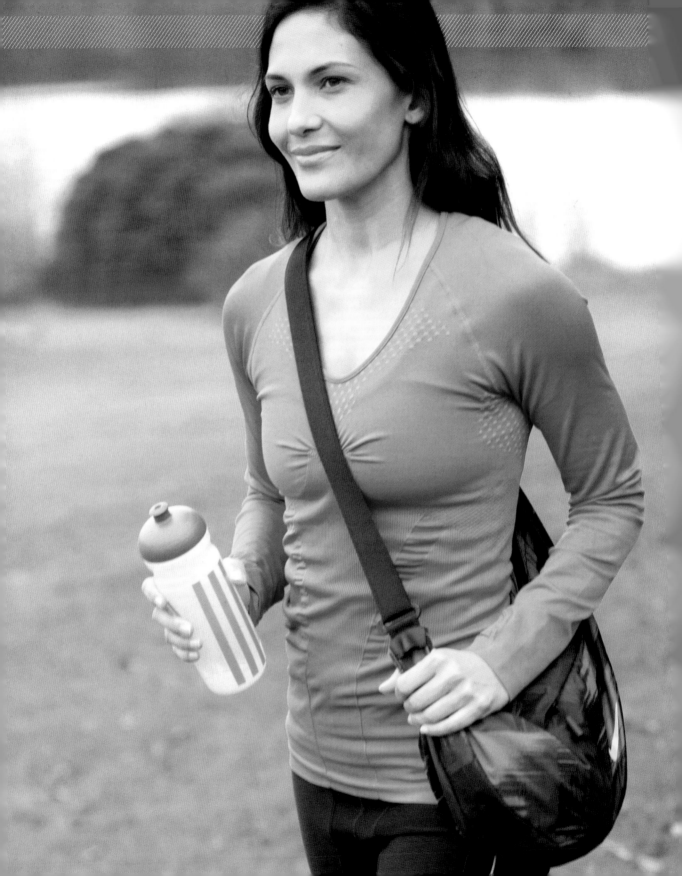

Events diary

Sign up for a charity walk and raise much-needed funds while getting fit at the same time

Nothing boosts your motivation more than entering a race or group event. From scenic treks and fundraising walks to competitive walking half and full marathons, there's an event out there for you! So get your friends together and choose one or more walks from our pick of the UK's best walking events for 2012.

Just Walk
MAY May 12, 2012

Now in its sixth year, this sponsored charity hike, over 10K, 20K, 40K or 60K routes, offers walkers the opportunity to fundraise for the charity of their choice. Pick whichever distance you prefer and take in the picturesque scenery of the South Downs in West Sussex while doing your bit.
Acrossthedivide.com

London 2 Brighton Challenge
May 12-13, 2012

This ultra-endurance event calls for some hard months of training to cover the 100K. Get a group involved with you as you'll need the support of a team to get through anything from 15-30 hours of walking. But celebrating with over 1,000 fellow challengers when you reach the Brighton coast will surely make it worthwhile.
London2brightonchallenge.com

London Stadia Trekathon
May 13, 2012

This tough one-day event will see you cover the urban landscape of London while taking in all the locations that are hosting Olympic events. Starting in Stratford and finishing in Greenwich Park, you'll enjoy the distractions of London's landmarks as you cover this marathon distance.
Discoveradventure.com

〉〉〉〉

Coventry Walkathon 2012

May 13, 2012

Enjoy a leisurely walk to raise funds for the British Heart Foundation. The route is 1.75 miles around Coventry War Memorial Park and you can walk as many laps as you like. So bring friends, family, colleagues and enjoy the friendly atmosphere – you can even enter in fancy dress!

Bhf.org.uk

Race for Life

May-July 2012

Since 1994 this event, the largest women-only fundraising event in the UK, has been inspiring women to walk, jog or run 5K to raise money for the fight against cancer. With a huge number of races on this summer you'll be sure to find one near you.

raceforlife.cancerresearchuk.org

Cambridge Oxfam Walk 2012

May 20, 2012

This event really has something for everyone. Choose from one of six distance options from four to 26 miles. The aim is to raise at least £30,000 for Oxfam's humanitarian relief work, so if every runner raised just £50 the target would be reached. It's not a huge amount and totally manageable if it's your first sponsored charity event.

Oxfam.org.uk

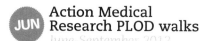

Action Medical Research PLOD walks

June-September 2012

Take part at any one of seven locations around the UK on this ultimate team walking challenge. At around 40 miles, a PLOD is not a casual walk in the park.

It's a long, strenuous overnight event requiring teamwork, stamina and coordination. It's certainly not for the faint-hearted!

Action.org.uk

Moonwalk Edinburgh 2012

June 9, 2012

A sister event to the already sold-out one in London, why not try this popular walk in the Scottish capital. Simply power walk in your decorated bra (the brighter the better!) to raise money and awareness for your breast cancer charity of choice. Choose from a full- or half-marathon distance in this non-competitive walk, which sees thousands of enthusiastic walkers joining each year.

Walkthewalk.org

JUL Sunwalk 2012

July 1, 2012

This daytime challenge, organised by Walk the Walk, is billed as a day out for all the family. Walk 5K, 10K or half-marathon distance (21K) around Battersea Park and make a real difference for vital breast cancer causes. The theme of the day is 'Caribbean Spectacular' so dress in your brightest clothes and enjoy the fun atmosphere!

Walkthewalk.org

The Prostate Cancer Charity Hadrian's Wall Highlights

July 6-8, 2012

Spend three days in one of Northern England's most scenic areas while you cover 25 miles along Hadrian's Wall on this guided walk. You'll only need a small backpack on this picturesque

route as your luggage is transported between your accommodation daily. There is a minimum sponsorship level for this so start collecting!

Prostate-cancer.org.uk

Kidney Research UK London Bridges Walk

July 8, 2012

Along a seven-mile route over some of London's most famous bridges, this is an enjoyable charity walk for young and old alike. You'll take in many of London's most spectacular sights, such as the London Eye, Big Ben and the Tower of London so make this a family day out to remember.

Kidneyresearchuk.org

Walk Ten Derbyshire

July 21, 2012

For a civilised walk, why not join the people at Marie Curie Cancer Care for a summer evening 10K at Chatsworth House? Stroll through the grounds at sunset, and don't forget your picnic basket to join in the festival-like atmosphere afterwards. Marie Curie holds similar Walk Ten events nationwide.

Mariecurie.org.uk

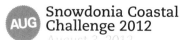

AUG Snowdonia Coastal Challenge 2012

August 3, 2012

Trek 20 miles along the North Wales coastal path with the dramatic mountains of Snowdonia as a backdrop. The course winds around an impressive Bay between the two Ormes (large natural rock structures) so make sure you bring your camera to remember this beautiful walking experience.

Timeoutdoors.com

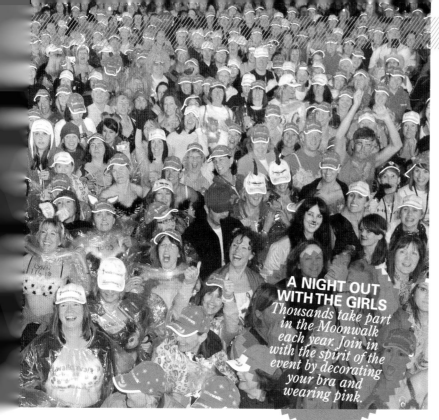

A NIGHT OUT WITH THE GIRLS Thousands take part in the Moonwalk each year. Join in with the spirit of the event by decorating your bra and wearing pink.

British Red Cross Peak District Walk

September 23, 2012

Enjoy a 12-mile walk along a section of the Pennine Way in the Peak District National Park. The route takes in Mam Tor, one of the highest points in the peaks, where you can appreciate breathtaking 360° views of the surrounding countryside.
Redcross.org.uk

Thames Path Challenge

September 29-30, 2012

This timed endurance event will see individuals and teams complete either 50K in 12 hours or 100K in 24 hours. The route runs from Putney Bridge to Henley-on-Thames with food and water stations at four points on the way. It's the ultimate test, but you'll feel a huge sense of achievement when you finish.
Thamespathchallenge.com

PinkPower Walk Northwest

September 30, 2012

This walk was inspired by the success of the PinkPower Walk in London. Set up in 2004, the organisation has raised almost £1million for both Breakthrough Breast Cancer and the Caron Keating Foundation. Join like-minded walkers for an enjoyable 13-mile walk.
Pinkpowerwalknorthwest.org.uk

 SEP

Alzheimer's Society Memory Walk Marathon

September 2012

If you want to do a marathon, now's your chance. Sign up to either one of these walks in Northumberland, Stonehenge or the Coastal Causeway in Northern Ireland, and you'll feel an enormous sense of achievement knowing you've covered 26 miles while raising money for dementia sufferers.
Alzheimers.co.uk

Spire 2 Spire Trekathon

September 8, 2012

A well-organised event, this diverse trek links two of England's most impressive cathedrals, Winchester and Salisbury. Covering a tough 26 miles, it's definitely a challenge but the support of friendly marshals and plenty of water stops will help you reach the Salisbury Cathedral spire.
Discoveradventure.com

Orange Autumn Challenge

September 9, 2012

This challenging, but enjoyable walk covers a beautiful stretch along the River Thames. Raise money for World Child Cancer by walking a 16-mile circular route from Little Green in Richmond to Hampton Court Palace. There is also an option to do a shorter 8-mile route and you get a free T-shirt when you sign up!
Worldchildcancer.org

Fight for Sight Carrots NightWalk – See London in the Dark

September 21, 2012

Now in its second year, this 15-mile route takes in some of London's most spectacular night time sights. Starting and finishing at the iconic BFI Imax on the South Bank, you'll enjoy seeing London in a different light while raising money for pioneering eye research.
Fightforsight.org.uk

 DEC

Festival of Winter Walks

Dec 22, 2012-Jan 6, 2013

Stay fit over the Christmas period with Britain's biggest walking festival. With loads of winter-themed walks on offer, from short ambles to challenging treks, you'll find a walk for you.
Ramblers.org.uk

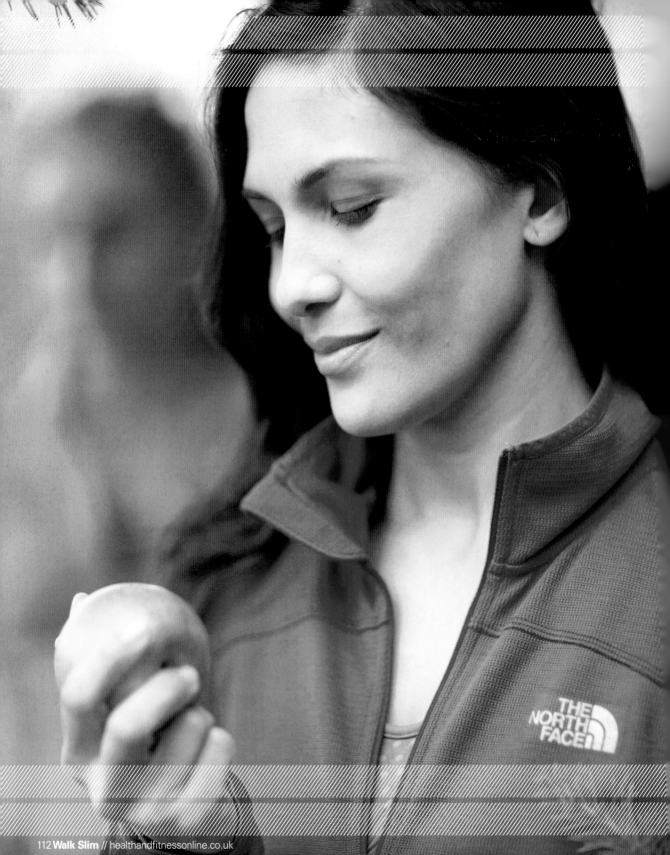

EAT SLIM

To get the best weight-loss benefits from your walk-slim programme, it's essential to combine it with a healthy eating plan. You can walk off weight but if you eat high-fat, high-sugar foods and big portions you'll struggle to lose weight. You need to burn off more calories than you consume to lose weight. However, the great news is that making the right eating choices can still mean having super-tasty meals. And you'll stay fuller for longer, feel less tired and get less cravings!

Eating a healthy snack in the morning and in the afternoon will help you avoid cravings.

Nuts and seeds are good sources of protein

Healthy eating

Follow these simple diet rules and you'll soon be looking and feeling your best

You're working really hard to burn fat and improve your health by walking – so why not back that up by choosing a healthier diet? Here are a few simple guidelines to help you slim while still getting all the essential vitamins and nutrients your body needs each day.

GO NATURAL

For optimum nutrition, choose wholesome foods as often as possible. Swap refined carbohydrates for wholegrains and avoid processed foods and ready meals as often as you can. Not only are they high in unhealthy fats and salt, vitamins and minerals are lost in processing and storage. Instead, focus on fresh fruit and vegetables, lean protein and low-GI staples. Where possible, go for organic produce or food with no or few artificial additives. Not only will you reduce the toxic load on your body, your digestion will function more efficiently.

PROTEIN POWER

Aim to eat protein with every meal – vital for growth and repair, it will also help you stay fuller for longer. Focus on lean cuts of meat, poultry or fish – a couple of portions of oily fish a week will ensure you get enough omega-3. Try not to eat red meat too often – no more than 750g a week uncooked weight – as recent research confirms the saturated fat content increases your risk of heart disease, while the sodium content of processed meats increases blood pressure. Nuts, seeds, pulses and tofu all provide good sources of

AIM TO EAT PROTEIN WITH EVERY MEAL – IT WILL HELP YOU STAY FULLER FOR LONGER

vegetarian protein, and don't neglect eggs – they contain all eight essential amino acids.

PORTION CONTROL

When it comes to a healthy diet, eating from all food groups ensures a balance of nutrients. The Government's eatwell plate suggests dividing your meals into 33 per cent carbs, 33 per cent fruit and veg, 15 per cent milk and dairy, 12 per cent protein and just eight per cent foods and drinks that are high in fat and/or sugar. If this seems too complex to follow, try visualising portion sizes like this: keep meat portions to the 》》》

SUPERFOOD SOLUTIONS

Some foods are particularly beneficial for your health, due to their array of nutrients. Here are a few of them.

AVOCADO

Avocados are rich in mono-unsaturated, cholesterol-lowering fats, plus vitamin E and folate. They're also a great source of vitamin B6 for vegetarians.

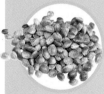

HEMP SEEDS

Hemp seeds are packed with omega-3, to help fight inflammation and joint pain, boost your metabolism and keep your heart healthy.

size of a pack of cards, pasta the size of your fist and cheese the size of a matchbox.

BALANCING ACT

Keep your blood sugar levels stable (and hunger pangs at bay) by eating three meals a day and having a low-fat snack in the morning and afternoon. To keep your energy consistent, aim to leave no more than four hours between eating – this will help minimise cravings for sweet, high-fat treats.

FOLLOW YOUR BODY CLOCK

The old adage of eating breakfast like a king, lunch like a prince and supper like a pauper is related to your body's natural circadian rhythms. Your stomach is most active first thing in the morning, when it functions more efficiently. As the 24-hour period goes

> **REDUCE YOUR CALORIE INTAKE BY 10 CALORIES FOR EVERY POUND YOU WANT TO LOSE**

on, it has less energy for digesting, and is more concerned with absorption and elimination, so keep meals light in the evening for maximum benefit.

THINK THIN

Use smaller plates – no larger than 10 inches. Research shows people serve themselves around 25-35 per cent extra food when using a large plate. Chewing your food slowly will help prevent you rushing your meals – which can lead to overeating. It also gives your body time to register that you are satiated.

DRINK TO YOUR HEALTH

It's easy to confuse thirst with hunger, so make sure you drink enough water to avoid piling on the pounds. Aim for eight glasses a day and it will help you feel fuller for longer too. If you don't like water, add a slice of lemon, or try naturally-hydrating coconut water.

WEIGHTING GAME

If you have excess weight to shed, research now shows the best way to lose weight consistently is to reduce your calorie intake by 10 calories for every pound you want to lose permanently. So if you want to drop one stone, you'd need to cut your intake by 140 calories a day. You might have heard that cutting 500 calories a day was necessary for weight loss, but the new research reveals this will result in hitting a plateau before you reach your goal. While the downside of this news is that weight loss will take longer, on the positive side, you're more likely to stick to your new regime, and keep weight off long term. »»»

SUPPLEMENT HELPERS

For those times when you need a bit of extra support...

A healthy, balanced diet should give you all the nutrients you need. But if you think your vitamin intake is low – due to a dairy allergy or not eating meat, for example – consider taking a supplement. For bone health, take extra calcium and vitamin D or to support your joints, try glucosamine and chondroitin. For extra energy, vitamin C helps your body absorb iron, which is needed to transport oxygen to your working muscles. Finally, make sure you're getting enough omega-3. As well as helping heart health, it's anti-inflammatory and may reduce pain after workouts.

SUPERFOOD SOLUTIONS

POME-GRANATE

When NHS consultants start recommending pomegranate to cancer patients, you know it's worth listening. Rich in polyphenol antioxidants, pomegranate is packed with vitamins and potassium, and helps reduce your risk of heart disease as well as cancer.

CHIA SEEDS

Part of the mint family, chia seeds are rich in omega-3 fatty acids, protein and fibre. They also offer high levels of phosphorus, manganese, calcium, potassium and sodium. Use whole with oats and other seeds in porridge, grind and add to soups and stews, or nibble on for a snack.

SPIRULINA

This blue-green algae is full of iron and vitamin B12, vital for maintaining energy levels and fighting fatigue. It's also a rich source of vitamin A and phytochemicals, said to help reduce the risk of osteoporosis and certain cancers. You can drink spirulina with fruit juice.

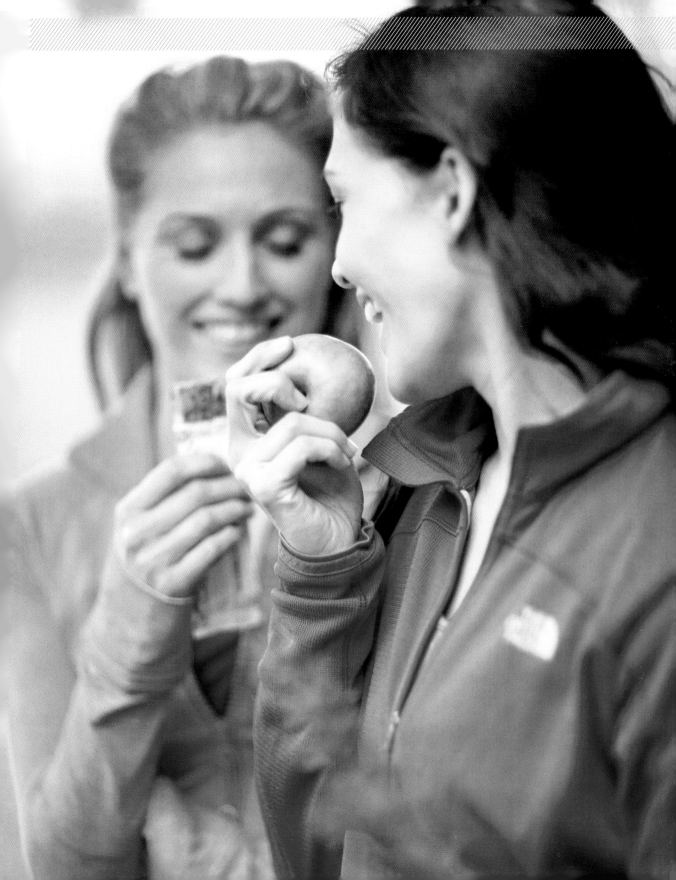

7-Day Diet Plan

A healthy diet doesn't have to be dull. This weekly plan has plenty of variety and tasty meal suggestions

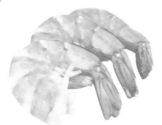

MONDAY

BREAKFAST
1 slice of wholemeal toast with peanut butter.
1 glass of organic or soya milk.

SNACK
1 fruit smoothie.

LUNCH
1 wholemeal pitta filled with tuna (in spring water) mixed with kidney beans, chopped spring onions and a little low-fat salad dressing or olive oil.
1 banana.

SNACK
Sliced red or green pepper with low-fat cheese.

DINNER
Prawn (or tofu) and vegetable stir-fry with wheat noodles.

TUESDAY

BREAKFAST
Wholemeal toast with grilled tomatoes.

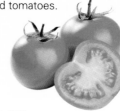

SNACK
½ a mashed avocado on 1 rice cake.

LUNCH
Small jacket potato filled with low-fat cottage cheese and chopped peppers.
1 low-fat yoghurt.

SNACK
½ an apple and 5 pecan nuts.

DINNER
Tortilla wrap (serves two) Heat 1 tsp sunflower oil in a pan. Chop 1 green pepper, 1 red pepper, 1 red onion and 1 courgette into large, similar-sized pieces and add to the pan with a little Fajita seasoning. Cook until brown. Fill a tortilla wrap with the veggies and 1 tbsp sour cream, 1 tbsp salsa and 2 tbsp grated low-fat Cheddar cheese. Cut in half and serve with any remaining veggies.

WEDNESDAY

BREAKFAST
Make your own cereal using porridge oats and adding a small handful of chopped dried fruit and seeds. Serve with soya, rice or semi-skimmed milk.

SNACK
Carrot and cucumber sticks with humous.

LUNCH
Wholemeal pitta stuffed with lean turkey slices, mixed salad and a little low-fat salad dressing.

SNACK
1 apple cut into slices with a little cream cheese.

DINNER
Steamed white fish with steamed mange tout, baby carrots and brown rice.

THURSDAY

BREAKFAST
1 boiled egg, two slices of toast and half a grapefruit.

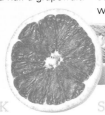

SNACK
Fruit smoothie.

LUNCH
Fresh soup with a toasted wholemeal pitta and a dash of spread or dsp of humous.
1 banana.

SNACK
1 toasted wholemeal muffin with ½ a mashed avocado.

DINNER
A grilled chicken breast or quorn fillet, with a baked sweet potato and peas.

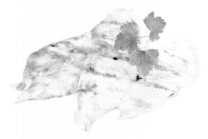

FRIDAY

BREAKFAST
Grilled tomatoes with scrambled egg on wholemeal toast.

SNACK
Cucumber and carrot sticks with low-fat cottage cheese.

LUNCH
1 small jacket potato with baked beans and salad.
1 low-fat yoghurt.

SNACK
1 banana and 5 almonds.

DINNER
Prawn and vegetable stir-fry with brown rice.

SATURDAY

BREAKFAST
Soak a handful of oats in low-fat yoghurt overnight, then in the morning add a chopped pear.

SNACK
Celery sticks with humous.

LUNCH
Avocado, ham and cherry tomato salad.

SNACK
1 oatcake topped with sliced banana.

DINNER
Casserole with beans, lentils, tofu or chunks of lean meat, served with quinoa.

SUNDAY

BREAKFAST
Wholegrain cereal with dried apricots, served with soya, rice or semi-skimmed milk.

SNACK
2 wholegrain crackers with peanut butter.

LUNCH
Small bowl of wholemeal pasta with some fresh tomato sauce and a little feta cheese.

SNACK
1 pear with a small handful of cashew nuts.

DINNER
Small grilled lamb steak or halloumi, served with cannellini beans cooked in sautéed chopped red onions and chopped peppers.
1 low-fat yoghurt with a handful of berries.

Drink up!

Losing just one to two per cent of your bodyweight through sweating can affect your performance. Here's how to make sure you stay hydrated for your workouts

As with any workout, when you're power walking, it's essential that you stay properly hydrated. If not, your stamina can fall and you may feel tired, light headed and suffer from muscle cramps – and that's not what you want when you're trying to boost your fitness and lose some extra weight!

The amount of fluid you need depends on how much you're sweating. Quite simply, the more you sweat, the more you need to drink. You're likely to lose between 500ml and 1 litre of fluid per hour, and more if you're exercising in warmer weather.

HOW MUCH TO DRINK

So much for the theory, but when it comes to deciding exactly how much fluid to replace while working out, remember that everyone is different. The precise quantity depends on several factors, including how quickly your stomach absorbs fluid and how much body fat you're carrying – fat acts as an insulator, holding in core heat and, therefore, affecting how much you sweat. Even certain medication can make a difference. Drugs, such as antihistamines and some blood-pressure medication, can decrease the amount you sweat.

One way to determine the optimum amount to drink is to weigh yourself before and after exercise to monitor your fluid losses. The Academy of Nutrition

> *ONE WAY TO DETERMINE THE OPTIMUM AMOUNT TO DRINK IS TO WEIGH YOURSELF BEFORE AND AFTER EXERCISE TO MONITOR YOUR FLUID LOSSES*

and Dietetics in the USA suggests rehydrating with 1 litre of fluid for every kilo of body weight lost during exercise. Alternatively, as a guideline, aim to drink 0.5-1 litre if you plan to exercise for more than an hour, or proportionally less for a shorter amount of time or a low-intensity workout.

WHAT TO DRINK

You know how much liquid you should be drinking, but what's the best fluid to drink? Plain old water should be your first choice. But if you're exercising for over an hour or so, you can choose an isotonic sports drink.

These contain a similar balance of electrolytes to that found in the body so can rapidly replace the fluids lost by sweating. They also provide a boost of carbohydrates. If you want to make your own isotonic sports drink, simply mix 200ml concentrated orange juice with a pinch of salt in 1 litre of water.

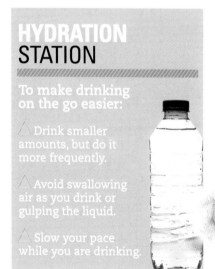

HYDRATION STATION

To make drinking on the go easier:

△ Drink smaller amounts, but do it more frequently.

△ Avoid swallowing air as you drink or gulping the liquid.

△ Slow your pace while you are drinking.

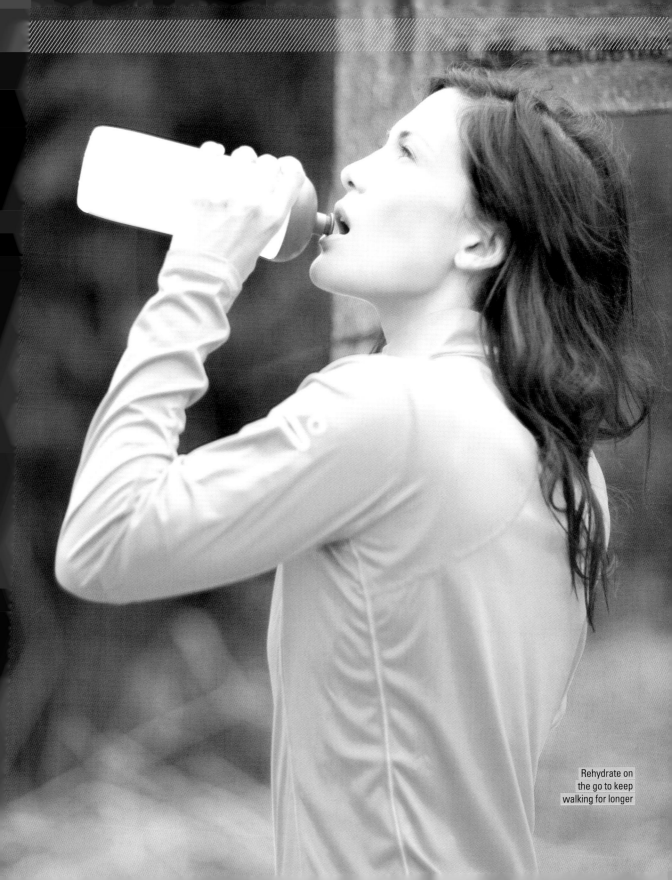

Rehydrate on the go to keep walking for longer

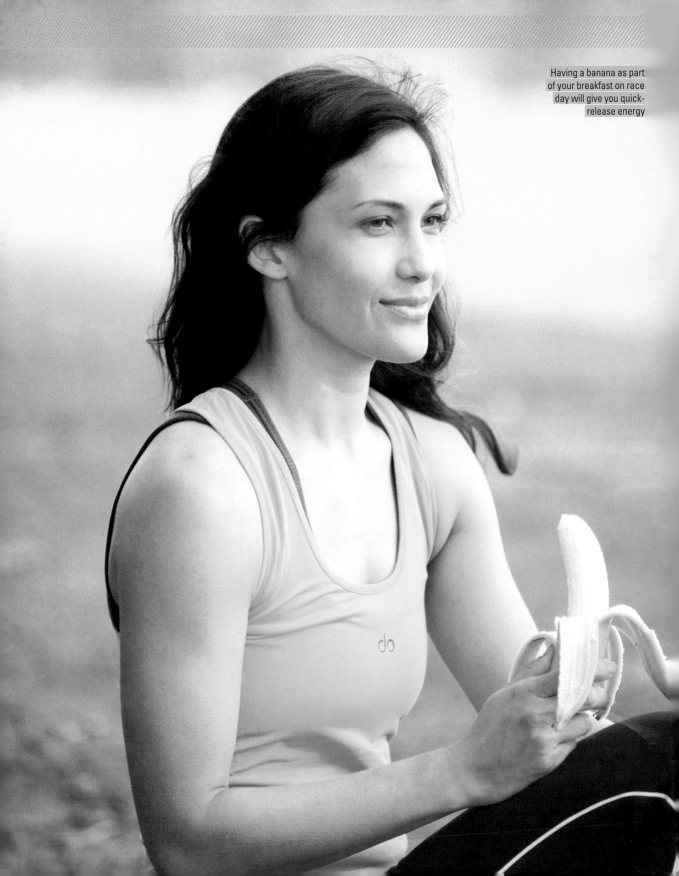

Having a banana as part of your breakfast on race day will give you quick-release energy

Eating for events

Make sure you have enough fuel to power you through your race

When you train for a big event such as a half or full marathon walk, you need to fuel your muscles if you're to perform at your best. Eating the right nutrients, at the right time, not only enhances your training and race performance, it helps speed up your recovery. Read on to find out how.

SIX WEEKS TO GO

As you increase your mileage ready for the big event, you need to increase your calorie intake. Your muscles use both carbohydrate and protein for fuel, so include both at every meal – aim for about 55-65 per cent of your daily calorie intake from complex carbohydrates such as oats and wholewheat pasta.

Protein is also vital for muscle repair, so ensure you include meat, poultry, fish, eggs or dairy (1.2-1.4g protein for every kg of your bodyweight) in your diet. If you're a vegan, you'll be able to do this with nuts, seeds, beans, tofu and meat substitutes such as quorn.

Keep your vitamin and mineral intake high – low levels can impact on your training. For example, low levels of calcium and magnesium can result in muscle cramps, and low iron intake can increase your risk of exercise-induced anaemia. A wide variety of colourful vegetables will provide the antioxidants you need to keep your immune system strong. Remember to drink little and often – hydration is vital for keeping your energy levels stable.

ONE WEEK TO GO

Start 'carb loading' to build glycogen storage in preparation for the race. Try to eat around 70 per cent of your calories from low-GI carbs such as wholegrains.

Decide which snacks you'll use on race day (see panel) and what you'll have for breakfast. Porridge, scrambled egg on wholemeal toast and muesli with banana are good. Don't forget to check your hydration levels by monitoring your urine (it should be pale and clear).

ONE DAY TO GO

During the day, eat light meals or snacks, and have a high-carb, low-fat meal in the evening. Don't eat anything you haven't had before – now isn't the time to find out something disagrees with you! Avoid alcohol the night before to help ensure you're at your best when you wake up.

RACE-DAY MORNING

Take plenty of time to digest your meal before the race – two to three hours is ideal. To reduce the need for toilet stops, avoid diuretics (coffee or alcohol), and don't overhydrate – have your last drink 20-30 minutes before you set off.

DURING THE RACE

If you're walking less than 5K you shouldn't need extra fuel, but for longer distances, energy snacks and gels can help give an extra spurt. They'll provide around 30-45 minutes of exercise so spread them over your expected time. Hydrate at around 500ml an hour, depending on how warm a day it is.

AFTER THE RACE

Have a snack within 30 minutes of finishing the race, as this is when your muscles can absorb the most glycogen. Go for a fast-releasing carbohydrate plus protein such as tuna or chicken on white bread or a bagel, a banana and 20-30g of nuts, or a protein bar (aim for a protein to carb ration of 2:1) and a small glass of fruit juice. You should also drink around 500ml (slowly) within the first 30 minutes after the race.

Follow this up with high-quality protein such as lean grilled chicken or fish with complex carbohydrates such as pasta, potatoes and rice, vegetables and a good fat such as olive oil.

ENERGY GELS

For a portable hit of sustained energy, sports gels are created to give you extra carbs when training or racing. Taken with or without water, some gels also help boost bloodflow and reduce cramp or muscle strain, or include caffeine to give you a mental boost. Easy to take when you're on the move, they're also designed to be easy to digest.

If drinking on the go isn't for you, carry some sweets. Sports jelly beans provide a mixture of carbohydrate energy, electolytes and vitamins B and C.

Directory

APPAREL

Adidas
adidas.com
00800 378 74737

Asics
asics.co.uk
01925 241041

Casall
casall.co.uk
01458 274557

Do Running
dounlimited.com
0871 423 2020

Falke
Falke-clothing.co.uk
01539 436655

From Clothing
fromclothing.com
01404 510518

Gore Running
gorerunningwear.co.uk

Gore-Tex
gore-tex.co.uk

Karrimor
karrimor.com
0870 838 7300

Kathmandu
kathmandu.co.uk
0800 066 5018

Manuka
manukalife.com
020 7371 7878

Merrell
merrell.com
020 7860 0100

Moving Comfort
movingcomfort.com

New Line
new-lineapparel.
com
01256 325844

Nike
store.nike.com

No Balls
noballs.co.uk
01638 570387

Panache
panache-lingerie.com

Reebok
reebok.com
0800 305 050

Rohan
rohan.co.uk
0800 840 1412

Ronhill
ronhill.com

Salomon
salomon.com/uk

Sheactive
sheactive.co.uk
0845 094 9434

Shock Absorber
shockabsorber.co.uk
0500 362 430

SnugBug
snug-bug.co.uk
01665 510660

Sports Bra Bar
sportsbrabar.com
0845 094 9434

Striders Edge
stridersedge.co.uk

Sweaty Betty
sweatybetty.com
0800 169 3889

The North Face
thenorthface.com
0800 328 0012

Vaude
vaude.co.uk
01665 510660

Zaggora
zaggora.com
07537 404575

Zocca
zocaactive.com

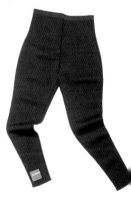

SHOES

Adidas
adidas.com
0800 3787 4737

Asics
asics.co.uk
01925 243360

Brasher
brasher.co.uk
0191 516 5780

Brooks
brooksrunning.co.uk

Inov-8
inov-8.com
01388 744900

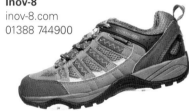

Karrimor
karrimor.com
0870 838 7300

Keen
keenfootwear.com

K Swiss
kswiss.co.uk
01458 449312

MBT
uk.mbt.com
0207 684 4630

Mizuno
mizuno.com
01189 362100

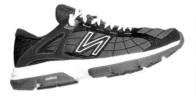

New Balance
newbalance.co.uk
0808 101 2828

On Running
on-running.com

Patagonia
patagonia.com
0800 026 0055

Reebok
reebok.com
0800 305 050

Rohan
rohan.co.uk
0800 840 1412

Skechers
skechers.co.uk
01707 624772

SpringBoost
springboost.com

ACCESSORIES

Gabel
gabel.it

Garmin
garmin.com
023 8052 4000

Leki
leki.com

Omron
omronhealthcare.com

Powerbreathe
powerbreathe.com

Satmap
satmap.co.uk
0845 873 0102

Silva
silva.se

Smovey
nordicwalking.co.uk
0845 260 9339

Suunto
suunto.com
020 3364 5723

Timex
timex.co.uk
0845 838 7573

1000 Miles
1000mile.co.uk
01923 242233

SUPPLEMENTS

Avogel
avogel.co.uk
0845 608 5858

Biocare
biocare.co.uk
0121 433 3727

Evergreen
evergreenhealthstore.co.uk
0845 2994 051

Maxitone
maxitone.com
01442 244330

Nature's Remedy
naturesremedy.co.uk
01663 741747

Reflex
reflex-nutrition.com
01273 303817

Solgar
solgaronline.co.uk
01442 890355

Vitabiotics
vitabiotics.com
020 8955 2662

FOODS

9 Bar
9-bar.co.uk
01490 412297

Beond
pulsing.co.uk/beond-bars
01452 728900

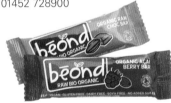

Bear
bearnibbles.co.uk
020 7183 0621

Bounce
bouncefoods.com
0845 838 2579

Bliss
pulsin.co.uk/bliss-bar
01452 728900

Cherrygood
cherrygood.com
020 7251 9924

Clif
clifbar.com

Eat Natural
eatnatural.co.uk
01787 479123

G.H.Cretors
ghcretors.com

Good Hemp
goodhemp.com

Hale and Hearty
halenhearty.co.uk
020 7616 8427

High 5
highfive.co.uk
01530 835873

Infinity
infinityfoodsretail.co.uk
01273 603563

Kallo
kallofoods.com
0845 602 1519

Nairns
nairns-oatcakes.com
0131 620 7000

Nakd
naturalbalancefoods.co.uk
0845 862 5340

Raw Health
rawhealth.uk.com
0208 547 2775

Rude Health
rudehealth.com
0845 465 7833

Trek
naturalbalancefoods.co.uk
0845 862 5340

The Village Bakery
village-bakery.com
01768 898437

ORGANISATIONS

Living Streets
livingstreets.org.uk
020 7377 4900

Race For Life
raceforlife.cancerresearchuk.org
0871 641 1111

Walk The Walk
walkthewalk.org
01483 741430

British Heart Foundation
bhf.org.uk
020 7554 0000

BOOST YOUR WORKOUT

For extra motivation to help power your way through the 4-minute workouts in this book, you can download *H&F* fitness expert Lucy Wyndham-Read's workout album *The LWR Fast Fat Burning Method* (£6.21) from iTunes and amazon.co.uk. The next best thing to having Lucy as your personal trainer, she will coach you through each move in the 4-minute workouts, giving you expert advice and letting you know how much time you have left to complete the move.

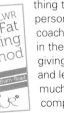

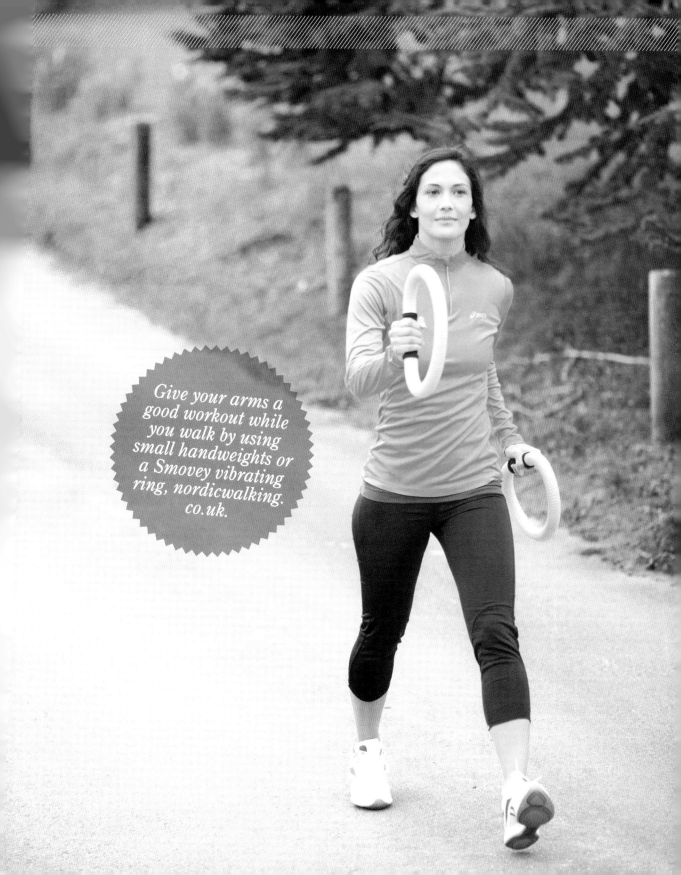

Give your arms a good workout while you walk by using small handweights or a Smovey vibrating ring, nordicwalking. co.uk.

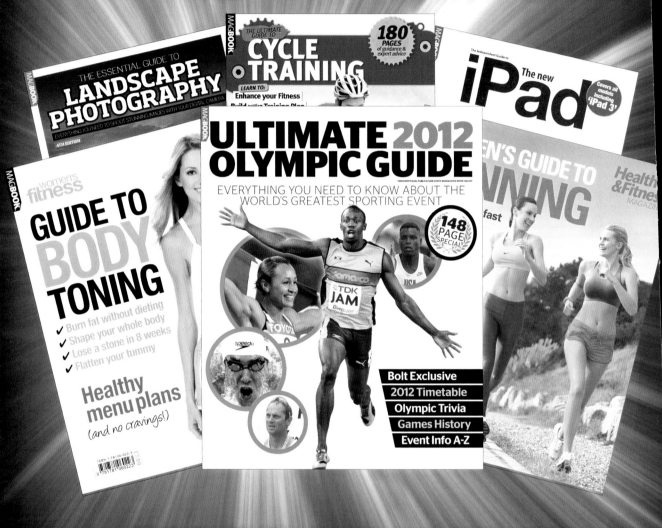

Health &Fitness

SPECIAL OFFER!
TRY 3 ISSUES FOR JUST £1

3 ISSUES FOR £1

Keep up-to-date with the latest trends in health, fitness and nutrition, and maintain your motivation by having news, in-depth features and expert tips delivered to your door every month!

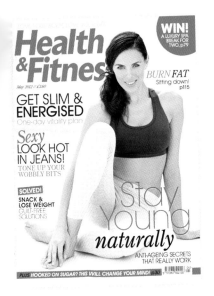

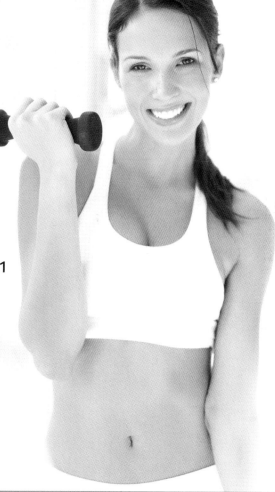

SUBSCRIBE TODAY AND RECEIVE:

- ☑ Your first **3 issues for £1**
- ☑ **30% saving** on all subsequent issues
- ☑ **FREE delivery** direct to your door
- ☑ **Expert advice** on health, fitness and nutrition every month!

Order online at **www.dennismags.co.uk/healthandfitness** or

CALL 0844 499 1763

using offer code: **G1206WW**

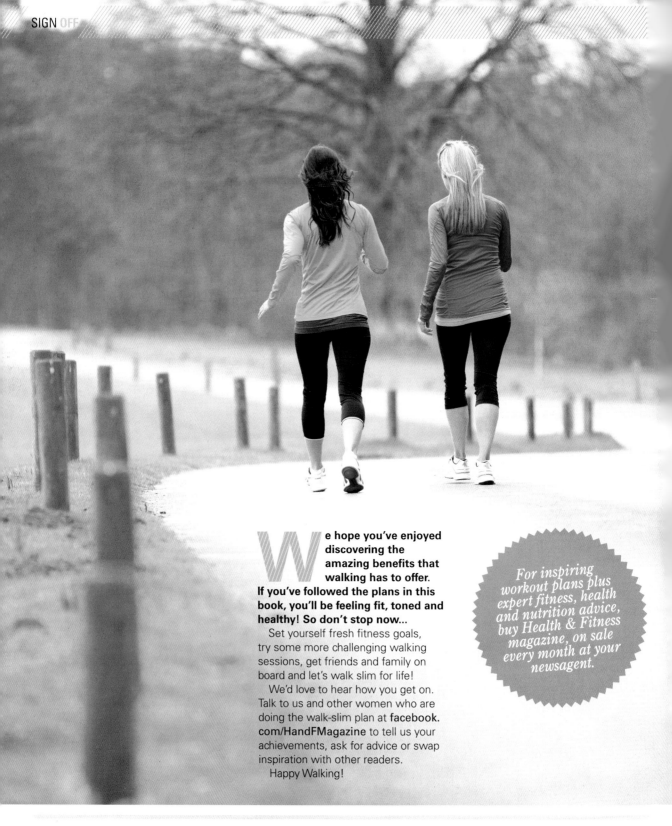

We hope you've enjoyed discovering the amazing benefits that walking has to offer. **If you've followed the plans in this book, you'll be feeling fit, toned and healthy! So don't stop now...**

Set yourself fresh fitness goals, try some more challenging walking sessions, get friends and family on board and let's walk slim for life!

We'd love to hear how you get on. Talk to us and other women who are doing the walk-slim plan at **facebook. com/HandFMagazine** to tell us your achievements, ask for advice or swap inspiration with other readers.

Happy Walking!

For inspiring workout plans plus expert fitness, health and nutrition advice, buy Health & Fitness magazine, on sale every month at your newsagent.